FREEDOM FROM INSOMNIA

Alexander (Sasha) Stalmatski was trained by Professor Buteyko and worked with him in Russia for 14 years. He brought the Buteyko Method to the West in 1990, working in Australia for six years. During this time he treated about 6,000 asthmatics and trained 45 Buteyko practitioners. Now based at the Hale Clinic in London, he represents Professor Buteyko and his method outside Russia.

He is the author of the highly successful *Freedom from Asthma*, also published by Kyle Cathie.

By the same author

Freedom from Asthma

Freedom
from
Insomnia

ALEXANDER STALMATSKI

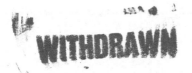

KYLE CATHIE LIMITED

Acknowledgement

The author and publishers would like to thank Anne Newman for her contribution to the text.

First published in Great Britain 2001 by
Kyle Cathie Limited
122 Arlington Road
London NW1 7HP
general.enquiries@kyle cathie.com

ISBN 1 85626 378 9

Text © Alexander Stalmatski

Project editor: Caroline Taggart
Text editor: Anne Newman
Illustrations: Colin Brown/Beehive Illustration
Diagrams: Ted Kinsey
Jacket design: Prue Bucknall

Alexander Stalmatski is hereby identified as the author
of this work in accordance with Section 77 of the
Copyright, Designs and Patents Act 1988.

A Cataloguing In Publication record for this title
is available from the British Library.

Typeset by SX Composing DTP, Rayleigh, Essex
Printed in England by Cox & Wyman, Reading Berkshire

Contents

Important Note

The information given in this book is intended for general guidance, and is not a substitute for individual diagnosis or treatment by a qualified practitioner or medical doctor. Always consult a medical doctor and qualified practitioner before embarking on any treatment. The reader is strongly advised not to attempt self-treatment for any serious or long-term complaint without consulting a medical doctor or qualified practitioner. Neither the author nor the publishers can be held responsible for any adverse reaction to the recommendations contained in this book, which are followed entirely at the reader's own risk.

Information about Breath Connection courses and practitioners in the UK, Europe, Australia and New Zealand can be obtained from the Hale Clinic, 7 Park Crescent, London W1N 3HE, tel. 0990 168146, or from the author, tel. 01523 192111. Australian readers can also ring tel. (02) 935 72236.

All *bona fide* Breath Connection practitioners offer a money-back guarantee of substantial improvement for every patient they have agreed to treat, no matter what the complaint.

Terms and Abbreviations

Breath Control exercises rely on a number of techniques which you will learn in the course of this book.

Control Pause (CP) – the major system for measuring breathing health – is described fully on pages 7-8.

The three levels of controlled breathing – **Gentle Breathing (GB), Shallow Breathing (SB)** and **Shallowing Breathing with Lack of Air (SBLA)** – are described on pages 42-46.

Maximal Pause (MP) – a powerful technique, which not everyone will need – is described fully on page 66.

The abbreviations are used throughout this book. For example a technique summarised as:

CP + GB (5 mins) + MP + SB (5 mins)

means that you should check your Control Pause, practise Gentle Breathing for 5 minutes, check your Maximal Pause, then practise Shallow Breathing for 5 minutes.

Introduction

'That we are not much sicker and much madder than we are is due exclusively to that most blessed and blessing of all natural graces, sleep.'

Aldous Huxley *Variations of a Philosopher*

'Now blessing light on him that first invented this same sleep.'

Cervantes *Don Quixote*

The famous words 'early to bed, early to rise makes a man healthy, wealthy and wise' make it all seem so simple. However, for the countless people who suffer with insomnia and other sleep-related problems, these words are nothing more than a useless platitude.

Although many of us spend about a third of our lives asleep, and it is apparently necessary for our health that we should do so, we still know very little of the nature of sleep and almost nothing of its purpose.

This book will take you on a journey of exploration through sleep, what it is, why we do it, and why it comes so easily to some people while for others it remains quite elusive. We will look at what causes sleep problems, and how we can solve them using Breath Connection. No matter how many other 'cures' or 'remedies' you have tried in the past, once you have gained control over your breathing, you will need look no further than your own bed for a good night's sleep.

CHAPTER I

The Theory of Breathing

It is a commonly held belief that nothing comes more naturally and easily as breathing. Yet so many of us are doing it wrong. In our culture there is a widespread assumption that deep breathing is good for us because it increases our oxygen intake. In fact, the reverse is true, and the more we breathe, the less oxygen actually gets into our bodies' cells. This is because the air around us contains a much smaller proportion of carbon dioxide than our bodies, and carbon dioxide is essential for each body's uptake of oxygen. So breathing too much, or 'overbreathing', results in a deficit of carbon dioxide, reducing the level of oxygen in the blood and tissues, and affecting the function of every system in the body.

What has come to be known as the Buteyko method, or 'Breath Connection', is a course of simple exercises designed to retrain the respiratory centre in the brain, thereby restoring healthy breathing patterns. Professor Buteyko, a Russian scientist, has developed the theory that much ill health is the result of the body's defence mechanisms trying to compensate for a lack of carbon dioxide. Deep breathing, he argues, is not a symptom, but a cause of many illnesses, ranging from heart problems to breathing disorders, all of which can and do affect our sleep. Retraining with Buteyko can alleviate a wide variety of problems – even snoring and blocked noses.

CO_2 – Not a 'Waste Gas'?

For over a hundred years, oxygen has been dubbed the 'gas of life', while carbon dioxide has been thought of as a 'waste gas'. In fact, carbon dioxide is one of the most important chemical regulators in the body, monitoring the activity of the heart, blood vessels and the respiratory system.

- The rate and depth of our breathing is regulated by the amount of CO_2 in our blood.
- When CO_2 is removed from the body in large quantities by excessive artificial ventilation of the lungs, the heart and circulation gradually fail and death results.
- The level of oxygen in the room where you are now sitting is 20 per cent. You would probably not notice if this level were doubled or even tripled because our bodies are 'blind' to higher levels of oxygen. Equally, you would be unlikely to notice any difference in your breathing were the level to drop considerably. (It is only when the level drops below 15 per cent, as at high altitudes, that you would be aware of the difference.)
- By contrast, a drop of just 0.1 per cent in the level of carbon dioxide can cause dizziness, palpitations, wheezing and a blocked nose.

Deep Breathing Test

Try this test to give you a better understanding of breathing:

- In a sitting position, breathe fast and deep through your mouth (as if you were running).
- After 40-60 seconds, or maybe less, depending on your general health, you will start to experience symptoms such as dizziness, palpitations, a rise in blood pressure, coughing and wheezing. When this happens, stop breathing deeply, close your mouth and try to breathe gently through your nose. The symptoms will disappear. If you try the test again, the symptoms will return.

What this test shows is that the symptoms are caused not by too much oxygen, but by too little carbon dioxide.

Hyperventilation

There are many conflicting definitions of hyperventilation, but from the Buteyko point of view, the key to understanding it lies in the word itself – 'hyper' means too much, and 'ventilation' refers to lung ventilation.

Most of us know from experience what happens when we breathe 'too much', or hyperventilate, say when we are blowing up a balloon or blowing out candles. We may feel dizzy and have palpitations and, depending on how long we are doing it for, we may even experience chest pains or lose consciousness.

Efficient control of our body's metabolism depends on maintaining a delicate balance between oxygen and carbon dioxide in the bloodstream. When we breathe at the appropriate depth and rate, this balance is undisturbed. But when we overbreathe, our carbon dioxide level drops dramatically. Paradoxically, while we are taking in more oxygen by overbreathing, it doesn't get to where it is needed because the lack of carbon dioxide causes constriction of the blood vessels, reducing the blood supply to the brain and the rest of the body.

Unfortunately, only acute, visible hyperventilation (usually anxiety-related) is recognised by modern medicine – a mere 5 per cent of all cases. The other 95 per cent of people who hyperventilate suffer from a variety of health problems, in which their breathing is not taken into account.

THE BOHR EFFECT

In 1905, Christian Bohr discovered the physiological law which states that when levels of carbon dioxide in the blood are lowered, the chemical bond between oxygen and haemoglobin (the substance in the blood responsible for carrying oxygen round the body) increases. Because haemoglobin will not 'let go' of its oxygen, it is difficult for the heart, brain and kidneys to get the oxygen they need. The result is that the deeper you breathe, the less oxygen your body's cells will get.

There are various reasons why we habitually hyperventilate, or overbreathe, and these may include infections, stress and medication. However, the most important reason is that we are trained to overbreathe. Western culture teaches that 'deep breathing' is good for us and yet this belief is responsible for no end of problems.

By breathing deeply we override the delicate reflex in our respiratory centre – a group of cells located in the medulla of the brain – responsible for the regulation of breathing. This respiratory centre then readjusts itself to a lower level of carbon dioxide so that a bad breathing habit develops and, in time, we feel that we are breathing 'normally'.

Back to Breathing Basics

Many doctors will say that it is impossible to relearn how to breathe – it is an involuntary process over which we have no control. Professor Buteyko argues that while breathing is controlled by automatic chemical and physical systems, it can also respond to our voluntary control. For example, we can hold our breath while swimming under water and we can increase our rate of breathing when we blow up balloons. Stress and emotions also contribute to our breathing pattern, and so does habit.

Breath Connection, the Buteyko way, teaches us to overcome bad breathing habits and to reset our breathing levels in a way that will greatly benefit our health and general wellbeing.

The Control Pause

Central to the Buteyko Breath Connection method is the control pause (CP) – the major system for measuring breathing health. This test is universal and can be used by people of any age, sex, height or weight, regardless of whether they are champion Olympic swimmers or elderly, women suffering from enlarged air sacs and wheezing.

To measure your own control pause:

- Sit comfortably in an upright chair. Relax and breathe out.
- Breathe in normally and out again, holding your nose after the outbreath. Using a stopwatch, count the seconds until you feel the need to breathe in again.
- Breathe in through your nose without gulping air.

The number of seconds you counted before breathing in gives you your control pause. The ideal is 60 seconds, but a CP of 40-60 denotes good health. A CP of 30 indicates that you are breathing enough for two people; 15 means that you are breathing for four, and so on.

Tips on Checking Your Control Pause Correctly

- You must breathe out when you check your CP.
- When you breathe out, make it a normal, relaxed and gentle breath.
- Do not take a deep breath before starting; keep a careful eye on children.
- Do not 'push' your CP by holding your breath for too long so that you then need to take a deep breath afterwards. You must try to catch the precise moment of your first urge for air.
- Remember, CP is not an exercise. It is a measure of your breathing health, and you should not try to make it look 'better' than it is.
- The idea is ultimately to increase CP – this will be achieved by eliminating overbreathing and not by practising CP!

CHAPTER 2

What is Insomnia?

'. . . sleep disorders represent another silent epidemic, much as hypertension was characteristic a decade ago. Neither the public nor their physicians understand that sleep disorders such as insomnia, narcolepsy and sleep apnoea are real illnesses with serious and pernicious effects...'

Wake Up America, A National Sleep Alert
September 1992

Insomnia, or habitual sleeplessness, is not a specific disease but a symptom of some other underlying problem. For many people it is debilitating, causing endless angst-ridden hours spent waiting for sleep and a never-ending cycle of anxiety and exhaustion.

Traditionally, insomnia is classified as transient or short-term if it lasts between a single night and two to three weeks, or if it is intermittent. If insomnia occurs almost nightly for periods of several weeks or more, it is called chronic.

It is widely believed that transient insomnia does not necessarily require treatment, since episodes are short-lived. We should not, however, underestimate this most common problem, and it is preferable to address the transient problem so that it does not become a chronic one.

To gain a better understanding of insomnia, however, we first need to look at sleep itself.

What is Sleep and Why Do We Need It?

Since ancient times sleep, and what happens while we are sleeping, has been considered one of life's biggest mysteries. Countless myths, legends and theories have been put forward, but we still don't really know why we sleep.

- According to *behavioural* theory, we sleep to suppress the body's activity in order to save energy and use it effectively when it is needed for survival. This suggests, indirectly, that sleep is a form of survival and as such, is not strictly necessary in today's civilised society.
- A *metabolic* theory suggests that sleep itself, or at least certain stages of it, are directly linked with the withdrawal of certain chemical substances in the body. In other words sleep is the result of metabolic processes in the brain or other parts of the body.
- A third theory suggests that the main function of sleep is to create the conditions for *growth and development* of the body, and especially its central nervous system.
- Finally, there is the *information* theory, which claims that sleep is needed to facilitate learning, memorising and storing information received during the day.

What we do know, however, is that sleep is more important to us than food – whilst we can survive for up to two months without food, we can't survive for more than 7-10 days without sleep.

INSOMNIA STATISTICS

- An estimated 100 million Americans suffer with some form of insomnia.
- 20-30 million Americans suffer from chronic insomnia.
- There are 17 types of sleeping disorder, 95 per cent of which are undiagnosed and untreated.
- A survey carried out in the USA in 1995 revealed that 49 per cent of adults felt they had problems with sleeping.
- Studies carried out in Oklahoma and California found that 20 per cent of all road accidents in the USA are caused by drivers falling asleep at the wheel.
- It is estimated that insomnia costs the USA $70 billion dollars per annum in medical bills, accidents and reduced productivity.

Different Stages of Sleep

According to the traditional point of view, there are several different stages and types of sleep.

- Stage 1 is a twilight zone between wakefulness and sleep, when we feel drowsy. At this stage the brain produces irregular, rapid electrical waves.
- Stage 2 is when we are actually asleep, but it is a relatively light sleep – you might say you were just dozing if somebody woke you. The brainwaves at this point are becoming more regular.

FOLK REMEDIES FOR INSOMNIA

There are almost as many folk remedies for insomnia as there are insomniacs, and many people believe that they can be helpful. Given that there is a considerable psychological factor at large in many sleep problems (see page 35), there ought, conversely, to be something in favour of a remedy that you really believe in. Here are just a few examples of remedies that some people find helpful.

- One cup each of baking soda and Epsom salts added to warm bath water to help remove toxins from and relax the body.
- A rhythmic noise such as soft music or a fan constantly whirring in the background.
- An aromatherapy massage with essential oils. Popular mixtures for insomnia or stress include camomile, juniper and marjoram; camomile, melissa and rose and sage, rose, melissa, and lavender.
- A warm foot bath before bed is said to help relaxation by drawing blood away from the head. Adding a little mustard powder is thought to increase the benefits.

- Stage 3 is a reasonably deep sleep, during which the brain produces slower and larger waves than those in Stage 2. Breathing slows down and becomes more regular, but if you were woken at this stage you might feel you had not really slept. Thoughts and images that pass through your mind are at the conscious level, rather than the unreal and jumbled level of many dreams.
- By Stage 4, we are in a deep sleep. It is difficult for somebody to wake us since the body is almost paralysed and unresponsive to outside stimuli. If we are woken at this stage we feel disorientated and it takes a few moments to 'come round'. This is non-dreaming

---

FOOD AND HERB REMEDIES

- Traditional herbal remedies for insomnia include aniseed, balm, basil, borage, camomile, fennel, hops, lemon verbena, lettuce, lime, marjoram, sage, savory, sweet cicely, valerian and vervain. Any of these can be used in the form of a tea taken about half an hour before bedtime. Use one teaspoon of dried, or two teaspoons of fresh herbs, to one large mug of boiling water, then leave to stand for at least 10 minutes, then strain, sweeten with honey if necessary, and sip slowly.
- Aromatic herbs kept in the bedroom in the form of herb pillows, bowls of pot pourri and sachets stored among your nightclothes. Sleep on a lavender-filled cushion or pillow.
- A popular American remedy is a drink made from a mixture of juices including broccoli, tomato, carrot, spinach, asparagus and blackberries. There is some evidence that it can help to induce sleep.
- Lettuce and celery are said by some to be mild tranquillisers, so a green salad with supper might be helpful.
- Cut up an onion and put it in a jar. As you are going to bed, open the jar, sniff the onion, then close it again.

---

sleep time (also known as 'sleep inertia') when the body restores its muscles, skin tissues and so on. The brain produces large, slow waves, as in Stage 3. It is at this stage that bedwetting takes place, sleepwalkers start their wanderings and snorers start snoring.

- Stage 5 is what researchers have labelled REM (rapid eye movement) sleep because during this stage our eyeballs make rapid movements. And during this stage – usually for just a few minutes at a time – we see and experience a dream.

SLEEP IN THE ANIMAL KINGDOM

Worms and insects have simple sleep, a form of non-REM sleep in which they are immobile and unresponsive, and their life-support systems are running at a reduced level. Fish and amphibians have a slightly more complex form of sleep involving some special brainwaves.

Almost all mammals have both REM and non-REM sleep. Bats and opossums hold the record at up to 18-19 hours sleep a day, and domestic cats sleep for around 12 hours a day. However, birds sleep for fewer hours and for shorter periods, some of them lasting quite literally seconds at a time.

There are not only differences in the length of time that animals sleep, and the type of sleep they experience, but also in the actual way in which they sleep. Birds can sleep while flying or swimming, and some birds and marine mammals can sleep with only one side of their brain at a time, while the other side remains awake.

We sleep in 90-minute cycles: light sleep becomes deeper, then lighter again and then we see a dream. Normally we spend half of our sleeping time in light sleep, a quarter in deep sleep and the rest dreaming. A typical night's sleep will be one in which there are four or five cycles of NREM (non-REM) sleep (comprising Stages 1-4 above), followed each time by REM sleep. Despite the fact that we spend up to 30 per cent of our time asleep dreaming, many of us remember our dreams only about once a week, and some people claim that they 'never dream at all'.

Dreams

Dreams can often be quite weird or fantastical like colourful movies in which we often play the starring role. It used to be thought that there are some people who dream and some who don't. In actual fact we all dream, but we don't all remember our dreams.

From the point of view of 'healthy' sleep it is better for us not to remember our dreams. If we are woken up during REM sleep we are able to describe the dream we have just seen; however, if we are woken just a few minutes after an REM phase ends, we will hardly remember our dream at all. So, if we do remember our dreams it means that we are not sleeping well: we wake up frequently and our sleep is shallow. Nightmares are this situation taken to the extreme: we wake up with a jump and remember them clearly.

Most dreams should just be a sort of background noise for the brain, and should not be regarded as a 'voice from another world' or the 'word of God'. More often than not they are a manifestation of unhealthy daytime activities –

FAMOUS DREAMERS

Many ground-breaking discoveries are said to have been inspired by dreams:

- The German chemist Friedrich Kekule von Stradonitz thought up the idea of a ring structure for benzene after dreaming about a snake biting its tail.
- Dmitri Mendeleyev, a Russian scientist, 'saw' the periodic table of elements in his dreams.
- Francis Crick suggested that DNA was a double helix after dreaming about it.

---

overeating, oversleeping, family worries, a full bladder – or they may be due to an awkward body position.

Dream Theories Through the Ages

In ancient Egypt dreams were thought to be part of the supernatural world, or messages from the gods. It was in Egypt that the process of 'dream incubation' began, whereby someone who was particularly troubled would sleep in a temple and in the morning a priest (called the 'Master of the Secret Things') would be consulted for an interpretation.

The ancient Greeks did not give dreams any serious consideration until the eighth century BC. Like the Egyptians they thought dreams carried divine messages that had to be interpreted with the aid of a priest. The first steps into modern dream interpretation were taken in the fifth century BC when the philosopher Heraclitus suggested that a person's dream world was created in their own mind. Aristotle later advanced the theory that dreams reflected a person's health.

The Interpretation of Dreams by the Roman Artemidorus (*c.* AD 150) is the first comprehensive book of its kind. In it, Artemidorus put forward the theory that dreams are unique to the dreamer, and would therefore be affected by occupation, social standing and health.

Biblical times brought a revival of the idea that dreams were supernatural. The Old Testament is filled with dreams, among them the story of Jacob's ladder, and many Christians held that God revealed himself through dreams. Later, Martin Luther was to claim that dreams were the work of the devil.

Sigmund Freud is the best known of modern dream philosophers. He held that although dreams may be prompted by external stimuli, wish-fulfilment was at the root of most of them, and our dreams are a reflection of our deepest desires going back to our childhood. All dreams, he claimed, had some important meaning. Carl Jung, a student of Freud's, believed that dreams are messages from ourselves to ourselves, enabling us to realise – rather than conceal – the things we unconsciously yearn for.

RULERS AND THEIR DREAMS

Many tales have been passed down the centuries describing dreams that changed the course of history. Alexander the Great, while involved in a rather drawn-out siege of Tyros in 332 BC, dreamed that he saw a satyr (*satyros* in Greek) dancing on a shield. His interpreters observed that this was a phonetic dream – the letters of satyros could be split to make *Sa Tyros* meaning 'Tyros is thine'. Influenced by this interpretation of his dream, Alexander the Great was spurred on to continue the siege, and was victorious.

Julius Caesar dreamed that he was having an incestuous relationship with his mother. The dream was interpreted as being symbolic of territorial conquest and, as a result, Caesar too was victorious.

At the age of 28 Adolf Hitler is said to have dreamed of being buried by a shell. It was at the Somme and, although all was quiet at the time, he was so disturbed by the clarity of the dream that he left the bunker and wandered into no-man's land. Suddenly, a shell hit the place where he had been sleeping, killing all his comrades. This dream, and his consequent avoidance of death, may have convinced the future Fuhrer and despot that he was especially protected.

Today, most psychologists seem to favour Jung's theory above Freud's, but there is still an enormous amount that is not known about dreams.

MODERN MEDICINE NAMES THE FOLLOWING AS TYPICAL CAUSES OF CHRONIC INSOMNIA

- Depression
- Stress
- Asthma
- Heart disorders
- Arthritis
- High blood pressure
- Allergies

Fast and Slow Sleep

There are many theories as to what fast sleep (also known as desynchronised or REM sleep) actually is. It kicks in 60-90 minutes after we fall asleep, and some researchers believe that it is needed for brain development in babies and for cleansing the short-term memory of useless information in adults. Sleep researcher Dr Hartman suggests that the main function of fast sleep is to restore serotonin – a hormone without which we would not be able to think – to its correct level in the body. In experiments, volunteers who were disturbed during fast sleep developed aggression and memory faults after 2-3 nights. A few years ago, scientists seemed to confirm the idea that a biochemical process that causes us to 'see' our dreams takes place during fast sleep.

Slow sleep (also known as slow-waved non-REM sleep) incorporates delta-sleep, and it has been suggested that this is responsible for recovery and physical rest. The most basic reaction in volunteers to deprivation of deep delta-sleep has been shown to be physical exhaustion. It is only possible to transform delta-sleep (see Different Stages of Sleep, pages 11-13) into shallow sleep by introducing noise and various irritants.

Why Do We Sleep?

While researchers know a great deal about how we sleep and have observed dreams for hundreds of years, there is still speculation as to just why we sleep (see above). Sleep and awakening seem to be two sides of a coin. Sleep is a rest from being awake, and we do one simply because we do the other; we sleep at night in order to be able to stay awake and function fully during the day (or vice versa for shift workers). So, that being the case, we should go to bed when we feel sleepy and get up when we wake up, say 8-10 hours later. That is not necessarily the case however, and our need for sleep will vary quite considerably according to how our bodies feel on any given day.

How Much Sleep Do We Need?

'The person who sleeps eight or ten hours a night is never fully asleep and never fully awake – they have only different degrees of doze throughout the twenty-four hours.'

Thomas A. Edison

A key factor in understanding how much sleep we need lies in realising that it is the quality and not the quantity, or the length of sleep that matters. A person suffering from chronic fatigue syndrome, a cold, flu, or low blood pressure might sleep considerably longer than the 'recommended' eight hours, but feel as drowsy, dull and irritable as an otherwise healthy individual who has had a sleepless night.

A commonly held belief is that by sleeping less than say 8-10 hours, we are creating a so-called 'sleep debt'. This is supposedly borne out by research studies in which volunteers allowed to sleep as long as they liked consistently spent an extra hour or more asleep. But imagine what would happen if volunteers were allowed to eat as much as they like, at no extra cost. Would they not take an extra plateful, or more? In the light of this analogy we can see that in the case of both sleep and food, 'need' is easily confused with 'want'.

The food analogy may be taken a stage further. In the same way that overeating is not healthy, 'oversleeping' is not healthy; neither can we sleep 'up front' in anticipation

---

SLEEP DEBT

In the 1970s, 17-year-old American volunteer Randy Gardner stayed awake for 264 hours (11 days) and 40 minutes. By the end of this time he was, understandably, very tired, sleepy and perhaps a little manic. However, when he went home to sleep he slept for the grand total of 13½ hours, then woke up voluntarily, felt absolutely fine and went about his business. Judging from this (albeit extreme) example it would seem that the idea of a 'sleep debt' (see above) is not something we need worry ourselves about.

of not sleeping later. We are expected to take meals at regular times, we are told that breakfast is the 'most important' meal of the day, and so on. But what of those who are just not hungry in the morning? Or those who wake up hungry in the middle of the night? And what if we are hungry at different times on different days?

Ideally, we would all simply eat when we are hungry and sleep when we are tired, but this rarely fits in with our work or social obligations. We force ourselves into a conventional schedule, despite the fact that we are all different, so that the physiological need to eat becomes a habit or a duty and something that we think we 'need'. So what is the answer?

OVERSLEEPING – A MATTER OF HABIT

British sleep researchers agree that although most people prefer to oversleep, in the same way that so many of us overeat, no more than 5-6 hours of core sleep – a combination of deep, slow-wave sleep and REM sleep, which is the most restful and restorative type – is needed for good health; the rest is a question of habit and is surplus to requirements.

Sleeping Less

In his book *Say Good Night to Insomnia*, Gray Jacobs suggests that in the same way that fasting can be a healthy, cleansing process for the body, so missing out on a few hours' sleep from time to time is not harmful. Many of us would, in fact, like to sleep less because we resent the idea of spending one third of our lives in bed.

Dr Jim Horne, a prominent British sleep researcher, maintains that from 5-5½ hours sleep should be enough for the average adult. He suggested that a gradual reduction to 5 hours might cause some drowsiness to begin with, but that in time most people would adapt without in any way compromising their health or daytime alertness. In trials, however, it was shown that after a while those people who did reduce their sleep time began to feel that they could not cope, and they returned to their original regime (as is often the case with dieters and food). Why should this be the case though?

Psychology plays a part here, in that many people are obsessed with the idea of 'proper' sleep and feel distraught at the very thought of lost hours. Again, it's the difference between 'want' and 'need'. But the psychological factor is just part of the problem. If we are to sleep for fewer hours, we need to improve the quality – or depth – of our sleep, and to do so means eliminating hyperventilation (see page 39). Once this is achieved, we can expect to reduce our sleeping time comfortably by 1-2, maybe even 3 hours, and

---

THE EXAMPLE OF YOGIS

If humans were 'designed' to sleep eight hours or more, you would expect that a yogi (a master of yoga) would sleep even longer – they have plenty of time to sleep. However, they don't even sleep half of the recommended amount. They go to bed, then wake up after half an hour or an hour. They then meditate for a few hours, sleep again and go through the same cycle. They also advocate staying awake for one full night every week.

go to bed only when we are really sleepy. If you sleep deeply you certainly do not need 7-8 hours to wake up feeling refreshed and rested. It is really only the first few hours of sleep that are vital in any case since they include slow-wave deep sleep and REM sleep (see page 13). The remaining hours could be said to be optional. (See pages 51-52 for a 'Sleep Less' programme).

Why Do We Often Feel Worse in the Morning?

Many people report feeling worse in the morning after a 'proper' night's sleep. This is because when we first fall asleep in bed our breathing becomes shallower, but after our bodies have been horizontal for a couple of hours it starts to get deeper and deeper, eventually (at around 3 a.m.) reaching a peak: hyperventilation. Asthma sufferers will then wake up with symptoms, eczema sufferers will start scratching, snorers snore louder than ever, and so on. Interestingly, a large number of deaths take place from 4-6 a.m. Growing hyperventilation as a result of prolonging sleep is the major reason why we should think about sleeping less, not more.

What About Sleeping Pills?

Many people who use medication to help them sleep feel genuinely scared about going to bed without it. The irony is, however, that sleeping pills are one of the most common causes of insomnia: getting off the sleeping pill hook severely disrupts sleep creating a situation called 'drug-dependency insomnia'. The patient is trapped in a vicious cycle.

Fortunately this is something that can be solved using Breath Connection techniques (see Chapter 3). The exercises not only deal with the problem of hyperventilation but, by raising carbon dioxide to a normal physiological level, have a sedative effect on the nervous system. On the first day of practising Breath Connection you should be able to take just half your normal dosage and, by the second day, cut it out altogether.

Apart from their side effects (such as drowsiness during the day), there are a number of very good reasons why you should not take sleeping pills:

- Insomnia is a symptom, not a disease, so that treating the symptom does not cure the underlying problem.
- After we have been taking sleeping pills for a while our bodies develop a tolerance to them, so that larger, more powerful doses are required.
- Some studies show that addiction can occur after taking sleeping pills for as little as three consecutive nights.
- In some cases they can be dangerous (for sufferers of sleep apnoea, for example – see pages 57-59).

A DELUGE OF SLEEPING PILLS

In 1973 it was reported by the sleep researcher A. Birah that 11,000 German pharmacies dispensed 21,543,000,000 sleeping pills (excluding those used in hospitals) – enough to encircle the globe 269 times over.

Sleep as Medicine

Based on the theory that sleep itself is therapeutic, sleep clinics or 'sleep disorder centres' have been established in the USA, Australia and all over Europe to cure various psychiatric and nervous problems through prolonged sleep. Their success, however, has been limited. Such clinics have also attempted to fight hyperventilation in patients with heart problems. Whilst recognition of the fact that hyperventilation plays a part in heart problems is a huge step forward, a vicious circle is created by attempting to treat it with sedatives: neither sleep nor sedatives will trigger a physiologically normal breathing pattern.

Sleep and Creativity

There is a myth that creative people need more sleep. Albert Einstein, for example, slept 9-10 hours at night and also had afternoon naps. But let's just take a look at some other great achievers' sleep:

- Leonardo da Vinci slept for only 1½ hours a day – in half hour snatches!
- Nikola Tesla, inventor of the rotating magnetic field, slept for 2 hours.
- Thomas Edison slept for just 3-4 hours.
- Napoleon Bonaparte slept 3-4 hours and sometimes not at all – he is said to have stayed up all night on the eve of Waterloo, for example.
- Winston Churchill managed on 4 hours sleep, as does Margaret Thatcher.

It would certainly seem, therefore, that we do not need to sleep great lengths of time to be able to achieve great things.

In fact, studies have shown that people who were allowed to sleep for 30 minutes every 4 hours during a 24-hour period were able to maintain an adequate performance during waking hours. Research carried out on soldiers, firefighters and astronauts also shows how they are able to function on small amounts of sleep, broken by interruptions, without impairing performance.

LONG SLEEPERS

According to Dr Hartman, a well-known sleep researcher, people who like to sleep long hours are suffering from either psychological or nervous problems: they are oversensitive, suspicious and overanxious. They have a tendency to depression and often admit that sleep is their escape route.

This may be borne out by a survey conducted in France: 800,000 people said that they sleep 8-8½ hours per night on average. The same group also reported that they sleep less when they feel well and happy than when they are depressed and unhappy.

Larks and Owls

The idea of 'early to rise' is popular in many cultures, based on the premise that a lot of people (larks) are fresh and energetic in the morning. There are, however, many people (owls) who hate the morning hours and do not find that they are productive until later in the day. After getting out of bed in the morning they feel sleepy, weak and irritable, and may remain so until midday. There is, however, very little known about what makes any of us the type we are. Our preference does not in any way affect our health or well being, although it can be difficult for larks and owls to co-exist in the same home!

LITERARY LARKS AND OWLS

- Tolstoy and Hemingway rose early to work.
- Dostoevsky, Byron, Flaubert and Balzac only worked by night.

Are You a Lark or an Owl?

Try this quiz.

If you could choose your bedtime, what time would you choose to go to bed?
Before midnight = 0
After midnight = 1

If you could choose your wake-up time, what time would it be?
Before 8 a.m. = 0
After 8 a.m. = 1

At what time of day do you feel most alert?
Morning = 0
Early afternoon = 1
Late afternoon/early evening = 2
Night = 3

If you could schedule the majority of your activities, errands and appointments for any time of day, what time would be best for you?
Morning = 0
Early afternoon = 1
Late afternoon/early evening = 2

A score of 0-2 suggests that you are a lark; a score of 6 or over would suggest that you are an owl.

Yawning

Scientists still do not know just why we yawn. For some time it was thought to be due to a lack of oxygen until an experiment was carried out in which people were given more oxygen, but the yawning did not decrease. Despite the fact that we yawn often when we are sleepy, yawning is not in itself an indication that we have not had enough sleep. Some researchers claim that it is simply a mechanism for stretching the muscles of the mouth and face. It can also help to relax our breathing, thus helping us to fall asleep when we are sleepy.

Interrupted Sleep

Continuous sleep is thought by many to be an essential attribute of good, healthy sleep. However, this is a common misconception. Many people develop what researchers refer to as an 'idiosyncratic' sleep pattern which is characteristic to them alone. It may feature interruptions and may differ greatly from what is considered to be a 'normal' pattern, but at the same time it may be a healthy one.

Some people, for example, wake up two or three times during the night to go to the bathroom, but go back to sleep without any difficulty and continue to sleep deeply after each interruption. They awake in the morning refreshed and able to function fully, without needing a nap during the day. There is nothing at all wrong with such a sleep pattern, although it might be an idea to drink less – and there is no need to fear dehydration if you simply drink enough to satisfy your body rather than your mind. In fact, one of the effects of breathing with a closed/taped mouth (see Chapter 3) is that you will not wake up in the morning with a dry mouth, so you should feel less need to drink in any case.

Some people actually sleep for as little as 4 hours a night but take long naps (up to 2 hours) during the day. Again, this is not a pathological problem, although cutting down on napping time would be good. Taking a nap in a sitting position, rather than on a bed or couch can help to achieve this without compromising the depth or restorative aspect of sleep.

Other people might come home from work, fall asleep immediately for 2-3 hours, wake up, eat, watch television until 2 or 3 a.m., then sleep for a few hours and so on. Again, if their performance is not affected during the day, this is not a problem.

So, if your sleep pattern is similar to any of those described above, do not be alarmed. Provided you are not waking up in the night due to pain, illness (such as hypoglycaemia), depression or stress, your sleep pattern is a natural, albeit unusual one. Idiosyncratic patterns are normal for many people and are not a cause for concern.

CASE HISTORY

Frank, a healthy American businessman, consulted me regarding his sleep pattern which was causing him concern. While he fell asleep without difficulty on going to bed, he would wake up around three hours later and read, watch television or listen to the radio for an hour or two before falling asleep again until the morning. He consulted his GP, who told him his sleep problem was caused by depression. The man tried to argue that he did not feel depressed in any way, but the doctor insisted, saying that it might be in his subconscious, and he prescribed a course of anti-depressants. The drugs did not help the sleep problem, which is when he came to see me.

Having heard his story I concluded that he suffered from neither depression nor insomnia and that, while his sleep pattern was unusual, it was not a pathological problem. I based this on the following: he himself did not feel depressed; antidepressants did not make any difference to the way he felt or slept; and he had a CP of 35 seconds. The man, quite simply, had an idiosyncratic sleep pattern (see pages 28-29), and his problem lay not in the number of hours he was sleeping but in coming to terms with it psychologically.

The Psychology of Sleep

In any assessment of sleep, the role of psychology should not be underestimated. Why is it, for example that some-times the more we want to sleep, the less we can? Why do children find it so hard to wake up and get out of bed on school days, but are up with the larks at weekends and during the holidays? And what about people who genuinely believe they've had a sleepless night, while in reality they slept for a good 5-6 hours? In fact, we all wake up for a few seconds several times a night; most of us do not remember these micro-awakenings, but some people, and in particular insomniacs, seem only to remember the awakenings and not the sleep. This may be due to the fact that they are shallow sleepers.

Interestingly, people will often say that they feel dreadful through lack of sleep (experiencing headaches, lack of concentration, etc.) but feel miraculously better on being told that less sleep is a good thing. It is thought that up to 50 per cent of people who believe themselves to be insomniacs are not, and they are simply brainwashed by common misconceptions as to the 'right' time and place to sleep. There are countless idiosyncratic sleep patterns that are perfectly healthy from the physiological point of view, but which people find difficult to accept psychologically, and it is here that the problems begin. If a person feels fresh and able to function well during the day, it does not matter how long they slept during the night.

CHAPTER 3

Treating Insomnia Through Breath Connection

Despite the fact that sleep-inducing medication is at the top of the list of prescribed medicines in the civilised world, insomnia is one of the few medical problems doctors treat without objective clinical evidence. Doctors seldom actually see the problem – the patient just tells the doctor that he has trouble sleeping and medication is prescribed on that basis. However, a patient's word can be very mis leading, as was seen when some Russian doctors researched a group of patients who claimed that they did not sleep at all during the night. Using a polysomnograph – a special piece of equipment designed to give an objective picture of the brain's activity by registering a whole range of physiological parameters during sleep – they found that patients actually slept for 4-5 hours. Their sleeping pattern was different from the sleep of 'good' sleepers, but they slept none the less.

In other words, many people who wake up 2-3 times during the night are inclined to believe that they are insomniacs, and rather than ask their doctor if this is the case, they just ask for sleeping pills. And some doctors (not all), in turn, prescribe medication without asking any questions at all.

Some researchers are unhappy with the term 'insomnia', believing that the word itself adds psychologically to the burden of being unable to sleep. However, none of the alternative terms used to describe sleeping problems is precise, and none really gives a full picture of what is involved.

Three Sleep Scenarios

- **You sleep short hours but feel fully alert and rested all day.** If you fit into this category you are not an insomniac no matter how little you sleep. You are simply able to function well on less sleep than most people, which gives you more hours in which to get things done (even if they may not be the most socially acceptable hours)!

- **You sleep short hours and feel fine for most of the day, but a little bit drowsy for part of it;** your performance, however, is not compromised and while you may want to nod off at some point, you can just as easily keep going. Provided that getting less sleep at night is not affecting your physical or mental output, it is quite acceptable from a physiological point of view and, if daytime sleepiness does become difficult to resist, you can always try the technique on pages 38-39.

- **You sleep short hours and find it difficult to get out of bed in the morning;** you may have a headache, you feel sleepy and weak throughout the day, and are moody and irritable too. This constitutes a genuine sleep problem and should be addressed using the Ten-Day Basic Insomnia Breath Connection Course on pages 43-46.

What Causes Sleeping Problems?

There are six factors that can induce sleeping problems:

1. **Diseases of the central nervous system** in which the parts of the brain that participate in the regulation of sleep and awakening are damaged. This causes real insomnia but accounts for only a small percentage of all people suffering from sleeping problems.

2. **Diseases of internal organs or peripheric nerves** where pain or other unpleasant feelings disturb normal sleep. This can be anything from asthma symptoms (or anticipation of them) to muscle cramps, and can deprive you of sleep for a long time.

3. **Neurotic disorders and functional disorders affecting the nervous system.** Sufferers from emotional problems (including mood swings), people who are obsessed with disease or those who have a tendency to worry unduly make up this group.

4. **Psychiatric diseases** can affect sleep centres in the core of the brain, causing very unusual sleep patterns. Schizophrenics may be asleep or awake regardless of day or night, experiencing a sort of sleeping fit. Those who suffer from depression also need less sleep than others, despite the fact that they long for sleep as a means of forgetting their worries, at least for a while.

5. **Changes of environment** such as changes in the weather, sleeping in a different place, entering a different time zone and new working shifts can cause temporary sleep problems.

6. **Drug abuse**, whether medical or illegal.

Psychology and Insomnia

When people cannot sleep, the problem becomes the focal point of their life and their major preoccupation. Long before bedtime the insomniac will start thinking about this difficulty with sleeping and then other health problems, financial worries and so on will work themselves into the equation. And then it'll be assumed that headaches, high blood pressure, muscle pain, feeling 'low', tiredness and many other symptoms are caused by a lack of sleep. In reality, however, most of these symptoms, including the insomnia itself, are due to a disorder in the nervous system (the main culprit being hyperventilation) and unsolved psychological problems (such as a family crisis).

Tackling Insomnia

There are two possible approaches to this. The first is to eliminate those factors that cause insomnia. This is the real treatment because insomnia is invariably a symptom of some other problem. The second approach, which is unfortunately more popular, is the treatment of sleeping problems *per se*, so that insomnia is isolated from the factors which induce it. To treat sleeping disorders which are, in fact, symptoms of other problems is like treating a temperature instead of, for instance, TB or flu.

The ideal approach would, of course, be a combination of the above: the complete elimination of the causes of the sleeping disorders and help towards normalising sleeping patterns.

Understanding Your Condition

Ask yourself the following questions, loosely based on a questionnaire developed by sleep researcher A. Birah, to help formulate an assessment of where/what your sleeping problems stem from, or indeed whether you have a physiologically-based sleep problem at all.

1. **How does your insomnia manifest itself?** For example do you have problems falling asleep?; do you fall asleep without difficulty but wake up too early?; do you wake up in the middle of the night and then find it hard to fall asleep again etc.
2. **How does insomnia affect you?** Do you worry about your health?; are you tired and moody etc?; do you lack concentration?; are you forgetful?
3. **How much do you sleep and has this recently changed?**
4. **Do particular conditions seem to affect how you sleep?** Possible causes include frequent travel, sleeping in a different bed or room, noises, light, smells and climate (high/low temperatures and humidity).
5. **What time do you go to bed?** Did you go to bed earlier/later in the past?, and if so why did this change?
6. **How long do you lie in bed before falling asleep,** a) when you first go to bed?, and b) if you wake up during the night? Has this changed recently?
7. **What time do you wake up in the morning?** And do you generally get up within 15 minutes of waking up?, or are you still in bed after 30 minutes?
8. **What do you do if you can't fall asleep?** Do you stay in bed, read, watch TV or listen to the radio, get up, or do something to try to induce sleep?

9. **Do you frequently recall your dreams?** And do you have a recurring dream or nightmare?
10. **Do you sleep during the day?** If so, how often and for how long?
11. **Do you take sleeping pills or any other medication?**
12. **Do you feel that crises or worries affect your sleep?**

What Do Your Answers Mean?

If you get up easily in the morning and you feel well and fully functional during the day, then your sleeping pattern may be idiosyncratic (see pages 28-29), but healthy none the less. In such cases, the problem is more likely to be psychological, a need-versus-want scenario (see page 20): you feel cheated if you do not sleep a certain number of hours at particular times but, in fact, your physical needs are satisfied and it is simply a case of convincing yourself of that. The programme on pages 51-52, designed to encourage less but better sleep, might be helpful.

If you find it difficult to fall asleep when you first go to bed, or if you wake up during the night and then seem unable to drop off again, it is likely that you have a real sleep problem, in which case you should follow the programme on pages 43-46.

Your answers to questions relating to recent changes should alert you to factors that may be having an adverse effect on your sleep. If you are able to pinpoint these you may want to consider revising these changes.

If you answered 'yes' to Question 9, your problem may not be insufficient sleep but lack of quality sleep (see the tips on page 47 to help improve your sleep).

Your answers to Questions 11 and 12 may lead you to

consider whether stress or other ailments are at the root of your problem. Steps may be taken to combat the effects of certain conditions (see Chapter 8) and don't forget also that many drugs, including sleeping pills, can take their toll on your sleep.

AMERICAN INDIAN WISDOM

In his book *Notes and Travels Amongst North-American Indians* (1870), George Catlin wrote: '…it requires no more than common sense to perceive that Mankind should close their mouths when they close their eyes in sleep, and breathe through their nostrils, which were evidently made for that purpose, instead of dropping the under-jaw and drawing air in directly on the lungs, through the mouth.' He goes on to say '…If he gradually opens his mouth to its widest strain …that man knows not the pleasure of sleep; he rises in the morning more fatigued than when he retired to rest, takes pills and remedies through the day, and renews his disease every night.'

Fighting Drowsiness

What do you do when you are overwhelmed with drowsiness but need to carry on? Try this exercise.

- Close your mouth and keep it closed throughout this exercise.
- Breathe out through the nose and hold your breath, pinching your nose with your fingers.
- Hold your breath for as long as you can. Count the seconds in your head.
- When holding your breath becomes unbearable, take

your fingers away from your nostrils and resume breathing, avoiding a big breath in or deep breathing in general. Try to achieve a calm, Gentle Breathing pattern as soon as you can (see over).

- Breathe gently for 1-2 minutes, then repeat.

This should alleviate your drowsiness, and once you have mastered the technique you will find that you can do it in public (say at a business meeting), secretly, without actually pinching your nose.

Note: This technique should be used only to combat sleepiness. It should not be used when driving, nor should it be used more than twice in one session or more than four or five times a day.

Combating Hyperventilation and Insomnia

One of the most serious faults in the nervous system responsible for insomnia is hyperventilation (or over-breathing) – breathing above our physiological need at any given time. Up to 90 per cent of people hyperventilate, and yet the condition is widely misunderstood, misdiagnosed and either wrongly treated or left untreated by many doctors.

In Chapter 1 we looked at the control pause (CP) – the system by which we measure our breathing health (see pages 7-8). The control pause, along with Gentle Breathing (GB, see over), Shallow Breathing (SB, see pages 41-42) and Shallow Breathing with lack of air (SBLA, see pages 42-43) are pivotal to Breath Connection. We will now put this system into practice.

Find your own CP using the test on page 8. If it is 50-

60 seconds, you do not hyperventilate. Your insomnia is not, therefore, breathing-related and Breath Connection will not help you. If your CP measures 15 seconds, however, you are breathing for four people all the time (possibly even more when you are particularly stressed). This means that the amount of oxygen reaching the brain is reduced, causing the nervous system to panic and making it difficult for you to fall asleep.

Gentle Breathing

To do this correctly your stomach should be more or less empty, so practise either before meals or about 2-3 hours after.

- Sit – a chair with a high back is suitable – with your back straight, looking slightly above the level of your head. Keep your mouth closed and relax.
- Relax your face muscles – lower lip first, then upper,

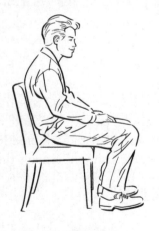 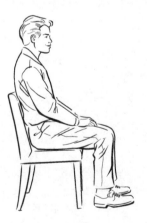

the wrong way to sit   *the right way*

then your tongue, eyes, and the rest of your face.
- Now relax your neck and abdominal muscles.
- Let your thoughts wander – try not to focus on them, but don't try and push them out either.
- Listen to your breathing. Do not attempt to change its rhythm or depth, but go with any changes if you notice them happening.
- Keep listening to your breathing for 15-20 minutes, or longer if you like, ensuring that your body, and in particular your face, neck and stomach, remain relaxed.

Shallow Breathing

You may feel aware of your heart or feel slight dizziness when practising this. Do not worry if this happens: it is not due to a lack of oxygen, and is rather like the effect experienced on coming out of a stale, stuffy room into the fresh air.

- Practise Gentle Breathing (see above) for 15-20 minutes, then put one hand on your chest and the other on your stomach. Watch how your hands move.
- Focus on whichever hand is moving more (usually it is the upper hand for women because they use chest muscles more than men, who will generally find that the hand on the stomach moves more). Then try to make it move less by taking in slightly less air with each breath. Everything else (your position, etc.) should remain the same, but the frequency of your breathing will increase.
- Do not try to slow it down and do not hold your breath after breathing in or out. Do not try to breathe to a rhythm, just leave it to your body. You should not feel

breathless practising this breathing; if you do, simply increase your breathing gradually.

Note: Do not confuse Shallow Breathing with slow breathing which can be deep. Equally, shortness of breath (often due to disease) is not the same as Shallow Breathing which is an exercise in breathing less.

Caution: Children practising this technique should be carefully supervised.

Shallow Breathing with Lack of Air

This is a very powerful technique and is a cornerstone of Breath Connection. It is the most effective and difficult Breath Connection exercise and can take time to master. You may experience palpitations or dizziness while practising, but these effects should only be short-term, and if you check your pulse you will see that it has actually gone down. Practise the following no more than 2-3 times daily.

- Practise Gentle Breathing (see pages 40-41) for a few minutes. Check your CP until the first difficulty (lack of air) and take a very small breath in – just enough but not so much that you lose the feeling of lack of air. Continue breathing in this way as follows:

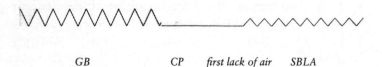

GB   CP   *first lack of air*   SBLA

In other words the lack of air at the end of CP is that lack of air you should feel when you are practising SBLA.

- Your breathing will be faster now and you should not try to slow it down.
- After about 2-3 minutes of practising SBLA you will find it difficult to keep it up, and may well lose it by taking a deep (or deeper) breath in. Don't worry if this happens, simply re-check your CP, catch your 'lack of air' again and try to maintain it for longer. Do not push yourself too hard, however, otherwise you will gasp for air.

Note: If after practising SBLA your CP has gone down it means either that you have not done the exercise correctly, or that you have overpractised. In the case of the former you should consult a Breath Connection practitioner; in the case of the latter you simply need to rest.

Caution: Children should not practise this technique.

A Ten-Day Basic Insomnia Breath Connection Course

Note: Before embarking on this Breath Connection programme you must stop practising any deep breathing techniques.

Day 1
- Keep your mouth closed for breathing all day (except when eating, drinking, talking, etc.) even when you are walking, running or playing sport. If you find this difficult you should stop and get your breath back

whenever you feel you have to open your mouth, or stop playing sport for a while.

- Sit and relax before breakfast and dinner, and breathe very gently and calmly, trying to involve your lungs and diaphragm as little as possible. Do this for 20-25 minutes. Check your CP before and after this breathing and make a note of the figures. The last CP should be the same or longer than the first if you did the exercise correctly.

- Practise Gentle Breathing (see pages 40-41) in bed in a sitting position (do not lie down) for 20-25 minutes – or less if you fall asleep!

- If you should wake up in the middle of the night, sit up and practise Gentle Breathing for 5-10 minutes. If you still cannot fall asleep after this, get out of bed and stay up until you feel sleepy again.

Day 2

- Before breakfast and dinner practise Gentle Breathing for 5 minutes then try to breathe even less, making your breathing shallow. Practise Shallow Breathing for 10-15 minutes. Try to forget that you have lungs and just breathe with your nose. Don't worry if your breathing becomes quite fast.

| 'normal' breathing | gentle breathing (5 min) | shallow breathing (10-15 min) |

- Check your CP before and after every breathing session, remembering that the last CP should never be shorter than the first.

44

- Practise Gentle Breathing before bed for 20-25 minutes. Try to relax more.

Day 3
Before breakfast and dinner you should:

- Check your CP and pulse per minute.
- Practise Gentle Breathing for 5 minutes.
- Practise Shallow Breathing for 15 minutes.
- Try to reduce your Shallow Breathing still further until there is a slight feeling of lack of air. Do this for 5 minutes so that you have:

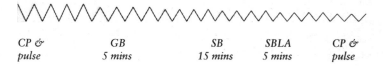

| CP & pulse | GB 5 mins | SB 15 mins | SBLA 5 mins | CP & pulse |

- Check your CP and pulse after each breathing session. Your CP should be up and your pulse down.
- Before bed, practise Gentle Breathing for 10 minutes and Shallow Breathing (but not Shallow Breathing with Lack of Air) for 10 minutes.

Days 4-10
- Before breakfast and dinner practise as follows:

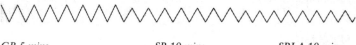

| GB 5 mins | SB 10 mins | SBLA 10 mins |

- Before bed practise:

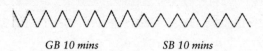

GB *10 mins*   SB *10 mins*

Note: If at the end of this 10-day course your sleep has not improved dramatically you may need to attend a Breath Connection Course.

Long-Term Insomnia

Breath Connection treatment can show dramatic and long-lasting results even in patients who have suffered from insomnia for many years. The most important thing is not to allow yourself to be distracted from the main goal, which is working on your breathing. Don't be tempted to try homeopathy or hypnosis, for example, alongside Breath Connection techniques. The breathing exercises are powerful enough to do the job on their own, and with practice and perseverance that's just what you'll find.

CASE HISTORY

Sam, a 24-year-old swimming coach, swims 100 metres under water with no difficulty. He sleeps for only around four hours per night, and yet he is in great condition physically and mentally – he works long hours and never feels sleepy during the day. This is because his breathing is perfect and his sleep, albeit relatively short, is deep and fully restorative.

EFFECTS OF HYPERVENTILATION:

- 1-2 per cent of adults (up to 5 per cent of whom are middle-aged men) suffer from sleep apnoea.
- 5-10 per cent of adults experience hypersomnia (excessive daytime sleepiness).
- 10-30 per cent of children and 1-7 per cent of adults sleepwalk.
- 20-30 per cent of children and 1-7 per cent of adults experience night terrors at least on one occasion.
- 30 per cent of 4-year-olds, 10 per cent of 6-year-olds and 3 per cent of 12-year-olds suffer from enuresis (bedwetting).
- 5-15 per cent of healthy people suffer from Restless Leg Syndrome (see pages 145-146).

Key Tips for Improving Quality of Sleep

- **Go to bed only when you are really sleepy.** By this I mean that your eyelids are heavy and you don't want to do anything but sleep. If you are not sleepy, don't go to bed – use the time to do other things.
- **Sleep on a rigid bed.** A Japanese futon-style bed is ideal, but not with a thick mattress; a water bed is the worst!
- **Keep a window open.** Fresh air, full of negative ions, is the best air to breathe. Deionised air affects the brain's respiratory centre, causing hyperventilation which, as we have seen, harms our sleep. House dust, cigarette smoke and air conditioners can have a similar effect, so keep a window open in all weathers.
- **Sleep on your left side, not on your back.** If you observe most animals you will notice that they do not sleep on

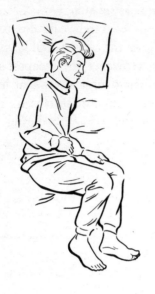 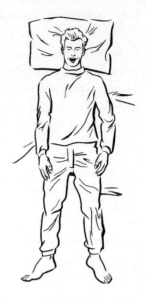

Try to sleep – or at least to fall asleep – in this position.

Don't sleep like this – on the back is not as good as on your side, and sleeping with your mouth open is certainly not recommended.

their backs. Dogs and cats sleep on their left side with their nose under their paws. Birds sleep with their beak under their wing, for the same reason, and horses sleep standing up!

Some people worry about sleeping 'on' their heart, but the ribcage stops us putting pressure on it, so it is perfectly safe. Ideally we would all sleep sitting up but sleeping on the left side in a foetal position is the next best thing. The right side is not as good as we sleep less deeply, see more dreams and get less rest. If you can't maintain sleeping on your left side throughout the night, at least try to fall asleep in that position.

- **Keep your mouth closed.** You will definitely get a better night's sleep if you do this. Over the years countless devices have been invented with the objective of keeping the mouth shut during sleep. However, the cheapest and simplest way to do it is by using surgical tape, at least until you get used to keeping your mouth closed. You might want to practise taping your mouth during the day, while watching TV for example, before leaving the tape on all night. Once you can do it for 15 minutes you can do it indefinitely! Many people believe that they always keep their mouth closed when they are asleep, but if you compare your CP in the morning after a night with and a night without tape, you will notice a difference.

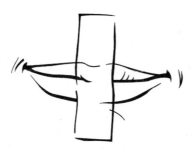

- **The less sleep the better.** The idea of sleeping is to get a good rest and be alert, fit and energetic during the day. If you can reduce your sleep time and still function fully, so much the better (see also pages 21-23).

Ideal Sleep

If your CP is very high you might experience a 'wonder' sleep. The scenario is that you start to feel sleepy between around 1 and 4 a.m., you lie down and you fall asleep as your cheek touches the pillow. You wake up thinking you have slept for 5, maybe 10 minutes, and realise that 3 hours have passed. You get up feeling completely rested, ready to face just about anything because your sleep was so deep and refreshing. Furthermore, you are full of energy right through the day with no feelings of drowsiness.

This sort of sleep is difficult but by no means impossible to achieve; it can be done by improving your CP through very delicate work with breathing and the respiratory centre. It takes time and perseverance but it is certainly worth the effort.

CASE HISTORY

Sixty-eight-year-old John came to see me complaining of sleep problems: he had no difficulty in falling asleep when he first went to bed, but would wake up a couple of hours later to go to the toilet and then be unable to fall asleep again. He felt that his problem stemmed from the fact that his GP had told him to drink a lot of water to prevent dehydration, which meant that he needed to urinate more frequently.

I explained to John that he could kill two birds with one stone by taping his mouth at night and therefore breathing through his nose. Breathing through the mouth is a major cause of dehydration, since a lot of vapour is exhaled, causing the body to dry out. So, by keeping his mouth taped, John would be less prone to dehydration, which would mean he could drink less, and not wake up at night to go to the toilet.

How to Sleep Less

As we saw in Chapter 2, and contrary to popular belief, it is less sleep that we should all be aiming for, not more. Try the following programme three times a day before meals in order to achieve shorter but better quality sleep:

Week 1
- Check your CP.
- Practise GB for 10 minutes.
- Practise SB for 10 minutes.
- Check your CP.

If you practise this correctly you should find at the end of Week 1 that your CP is higher than 20 seconds. This should enable you to decrease your sleep by at least one hour without compromising your output during the day. If your CP does not increase after the first week you should consider consulting a qualified Breath Connection practitioner.

Week 2
Assuming that all went well in Week 1, you may like to decrease your sleep time further. Repeat the routine for Week 1, but increase the Shallow Breathing to 20 minutes per session. Your CP should again be higher. To go further still, move on to Week 3.

Week 3
The following exercise may be done before breakfast and before bed, and can benefit both your sleep and your health in general.

- Check your CP.
- Practise GB (10 mins) + SB (10 mins) + SBLA (10 mins)
- Check your CP.

Key Points in the Prevention of Insomnia

- **Get up at the same time every morning.** Try to do this regardless of how much sleep you have had during the night.
- **Avoid sleep during the day.** Sleeping in the daytime can spoil a night's sleep. Resist drowsiness using the technique on pages 38-39, but if you are still sleepy after that a short nap may be the only answer (in the same way that we sometimes need a 'snack' to allay our hunger).
- **Try not to worry if you have not slept well for a night or two.** Don't dwell on 'lost' sleep, just try to accept it and move on.
- **Try not to worry that you will not be able to fall asleep.** The more you worry, the more difficult you will find it to fall asleep. We all have to sleep, and sooner or later your body will make you sleepy and simply 'switch you off' for a few hours.
- **Avoid sleeping medication.** Taking sleeping pills, even for no more than a few nights, can cause addiction and lead to a diagnosis of drug-dependent insomnia (see page 23).
- **Avoid big meals, caffeine, alcohol and smoking before bed.**
- **Avoid hyperventilation and all situations that cause it.** They may include breathing through the mouth, deep-breathing exercises, overeating, oversleeping, lack of

fresh air. Stress is also a trigger and, while we all need a certain amount of 'healthy' stress in our lives, we must not allow it to become distress.

CHAPTER 4

Sleep-Related Problems and their Treatment

Snoring

Snoring is one of the most common sleep-related problems, causing discomfort and disturbances not only for the snorers themselves but for their partners too – who can say how many relationships have been put to the test by this irritating and sometimes ear-splitting phenomenon?

Snoring is a typical manifestation of hyperventilation (see pages 5-7), but its cause is still unknown. It is often explained as a sound caused by vibrations of the soft parts of the mouth and throat area, but this is really a description and not an explanation. It has been suggested that in the distant past our ancestors were most vulnerable to enemies when they were asleep, and that snoring may have served a useful purpose in keeping them at bay.

In the 1980s a four-year study on chronic snorers was conducted by Finnish scientists. Among their findings was the fact that more snorers than non-snorers suffered from high blood pressure. A Japanese study carried out in 1996 found that a rise in blood pressure seemed to follow a poor night's sleep.

Snoring can be exacerbated by sleeping on the back, excessive body weight, cold, flu, a blocked nose, polyps, adenoids, or a heavy meal or too much alcohol before bed. While you may address these contributory factors, you must also treat hyperventilation as a cause, rather than snoring as a noise. That's why 'breathe-easy' patches, and operations on polyps, the soft palate and so on are not the answer. They may be successful in the short term, but cause more health problems in the long run. By using these methods you simply 'shoot the messenger' – snoring – without even bothering to read the actual message.

Who Snores?

- While 20 per cent of men under 30 snore, only 5 per cent of women do.
- 40 per cent of women and 60 per cent of men aged 50 and over snore.
- 5 per cent of people who snore go on to develop sleep apnoea (see pages 57-59), but 95 per cent of cases are undiagnosed.
- In 1993 a Swede, K. Valkert, became the proud holder of the Loudest Snorer record when he hit a deafening and quite astonishing 93 decibels – about the noise level of a kalashnikov!

What to Do

In 1915 a Mr George Little of Pennsylvania wrote to *House-wife Magazine*, desperately seeking advice on how to stop snoring in order to save his marriage. The printed reply was from a Mrs D. P., who wrote: 'Did you know that Indians never snore? . . . The secret is that Indians teach their children to sleep with a closed mouth from a young age.'

Indeed George Catlin, author of *Notes and Travels Amongst the North-American Indians* (1870), made the same observation. He visited 150 tribes ('more than two million souls') and noted a striking difference between the health of these people and that of 'civilised' society: no stillbirths, hardly any lung or bronchial problems, and strong and beautiful teeth.

To stop snoring you must deal with hyperventilation. The first three of the steps given below should be enough to help 75 per cent of snorers; the remaining 25 per cent will probably need step 4 as well:

- Go to bed only when you are sleepy.
- Tape your mouth with surgical tape (see page 49).
- Sleep on your left side – if not on your front.
- Practise Gentle Breathing and Shallow Breathing for 10 minutes each before you go to bed.

Note: If you suffer from both snoring and insomnia, practise the Basic Insomnia Course (see pages 43-46).

OLD WIVES' SNORING REMEDIES

- Place salt in the mouth and keep it there until it has dissolved.
- Sleep on a high pile of pillows.
- Bite your pillow for as long as you can.
- Prince Charles has been said to advocate putting toothpaste in the nostrils before going to bed.

HOW BADLY DO YOU SNORE?

The following questions should help you to form an assessment of just how bad a snoring problem you have:

1. Do people tell you that you snore?
2. Is your partner disturbed by your snoring?
3. Does it disturb people in neighbouring rooms?
4. Has your snoring become progressively worse?
5. Do you only snore when you sleep on your back?
6. Do you snore in all sleeping positions?
7. Have you been told that you stop breathing between snores?
8. Does your snoring cause you to awaken suddenly?
9. Do you snore at night and feel sleepy during the day?
10. Do you snore at night and have high blood pressure?

Evaluating your answers

If you answered 'yes' to Questions 1, 2, 3 and 4 your snoring is affecting your personal/family relationships which can cause stress (see pages 146-148), and related problems.

If you answered 'yes' to question 5, you might find that sleeping on your left side will help. This is the position that everyone should adopt in any case, regardless of whether or not they snore (see pages 47-48).

If you answered 'yes' to Questions 4, 6, 7, 8, 9 and 10 you are probably suffering from sleep apnoea which needs prompt attention (see below).

Sleep Apnoea

Snoring causes great embarrassment to many adults, and can also make children a target for ridicule and bullying. However, these become minor problems in the face of sleep apnoea, of which snoring is the first stage.

Sleep apnoea is a condition in which breathing is temporarily suspended during sleep. What happens to sufferers is this:

- They hyperventilate.
- They hyperventilate more in bed when the body is horizontal.
- Their carbon dioxide level drops due to the Bohr effect (see page 6) and causes spontaneous cessation of breathing.

People who suffer from sleep apnoea are more susceptible than others to:

- Heart disease.
- High blood pressure and pulmonary hypertension.
- Strokes.
- Problems with concentration and memory.

Sleep apnoea is as yet a largely undiagnosed problem in modern medicine, not least because many of the people who suffer from it are unaware of their condition. They stop breathing for say 40-60 seconds and wake up frequently at night (although they don't remember doing so) during both the REM and non-REM stages of sleep. Non-REM sleep plays an important role in maintaining a healthy neurochemical balance. It is also the deepest stage of sleep, which means that sufferers experience daytime fatigue having been deprived of their most refreshing sleep, and live with a growing dread of the nights to come.

Often sufferers are referred to sleep clinics where they are prescribed a CPAP (Continuous Positive Air Pressure) machine – a small air pump which applies constant pressure to keep the air passages open. It does help to begin with at least, but because it addresses the symptoms and not the cause of the problem, it can only ever provide short-term relief.

In fact, to a certain extent, apnoea is a normal part of every breathing cycle: we 'stop' breathing thousands of times a day, and hundreds of times during a normal night's sleep:

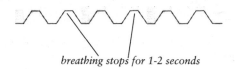

breathing stops for 1-2 seconds

In the case of snoring or deep breathing, however, breathing patterns change, apnoea becomes longer and the level of oxygen drops and problems arise.

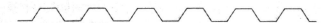

So as we have seen above, the cause of sleep apnoea is hyperventilation and neither surgical reshaping of the soft palate nor the use of CPAP machines will help in the long term. In fact, using CPAP pumps actually increases hyperventilation, so that it becomes rather like treating diabetes with sugar! If you suspect that you suffer from sleep apnoea it is not, therefore, advisable to attend a sleep clinic. If you have already been diagnosed and been prescribed a CPAP pump, you should try to stop using it as soon as possible.

Disadvantages of Using a CPAP Machine

A CPAP machine does seem to have some positive effects to begin with, but it generally only provides short-term relief and in the meantime it can cause any or all of the following:

- Headaches on waking up.
- Nosebleeds.
- Irritation of the eyes.
- Ear infections.
- Rifts between partners since its humming can be disturbing.
- Increased hyperventilation since using it generally means sleeping on the back.

With all this in mind it is indeed a sad thought that up to 200,000 people in the USA alone are using a CPAP every night.

CASE HISTORY

Forty-four-year-old Al is the manager of a large electronics company. He became a heavy snorer around 10 years ago and his wife noticed that the problem seemed to be worsening along with his increasing weight – he was 130kg (21 stone). Al felt that he slept well, he functioned well at work and did not feel unhealthy in any way. However, for the sake of his family, he underwent a surgical procedure to solve the snoring problem. Which it actually did at least for a while.

Then the snoring returned and his wife also noticed that his breathing stopped periodically. Soon he began to complain of palpitations, headaches in the morning and drowsiness during the day. His doctor referred him to a sleep clinic, where his problem was diagnosed as sleep apnoea. He was given a CPAP machine (see page 60), which seemed to work, although he did have some nosebleeds and a heavy dull feeling in his head. However, the drowsiness soon returned and Al would fall asleep in business meetings or at restaurants. His doctor increased the air pressure in his machine.

The final straw came in 1996 when Al fell asleep at the wheel of his car and narrowly avoided an accident. This is when he came to me. His CP was 5 seconds, his pulse 120, and he even fell asleep between questions. I told Al to tape his mouth before bed, to sleep in a sitting position and to fall asleep without using the machine, using it only if he woke up and felt that he had to. On the first night Al woke up after three hours and put the machine on. The second and third nights were the same, but on the fourth, he forgot to use it – he woke up, but went back to sleep on his own. Within two weeks he had stopped using the machine altogether. His breathing at night was much better, and his CP rose to 15 seconds.

Sleep Apnoea Treatment Plan

Day 1

- Follow the treatment as outlined for snoring on page 56.
- At bedtime tape your mouth (see page 49), and set your alarm clock to wake you after three hours' sleep i.e. if you go to bed at midnight, you should set your alarm for 3 a.m. If you have been using a CPAP machine for more than a few months you should set the alarm for two, not three hours' time and try to fall asleep without it.
- Sit up when your alarm goes off and listen to your breathing.
- If you are satisfied your breathing is not heavy and you are not in any way breathless, go straight back to sleep.
- If your breathing is deep and heavy, practise Shallow Breathing (see pages 41-42) for 10 minutes, then Gentle Breathing for 5 minutes and check your CP. Then set the alarm for 2-3 hours later and go to sleep. If you do not feel sleepy get out of bed, and go back only when you are ready to sleep.
- If you feel that you need to use the CPAP machine at any time after you wake up you may do so.

Day 2

- Before breakfast practise Shallow Breathing for 10 minutes, then Gentle Breathing for 5 minutes and check your CP.
- Whenever you feel tired or sleepy during the day you should:

- Stop what you are doing.
- Change the position of your body.
- Wash your face with cold water.
- If none of this works, take a short nap (20-30 minutes) in a sitting position – do not lie down.
- Repeat the Shallow Breathing and Gentle Breathing routine before dinner and bed. Then:
    - If you had to use the CPAP machine the first night, follow the same routine with the alarm clock (every 2 hours).
    - If you did not use the CPAP but discovered that your breathing was heavy, or you could not keep the tape on, set the alarm just once, for 3 a.m.
    - If you managed to keep the tape on, had no trouble the first night and felt reasonably fresh all day you do not need to set the alarm. However you must still keep the tape on and continue with the Shallow Breathing and Gentle Breathing routine described on Day 1.

Day 3
- If you experienced significant improvements in your sleep, simply repeat the Shallow Breathing and Gentle Breathing routine described on Day 1.
- If you still had to use the CPAP machine, keep setting the alarm clock as for Days 1 and 2.

Day 4
- If, by the end of Day 3, you still have not achieved results, practise the following exercise which is more powerful, involving, as it does, the Maximal Pause (see over):

SB (5 mins) + MP (= CP + 5 secs) + SB (10 mins) + MP
(= CP + 10 secs) + SB (10 mins)

Remember to check your CP at the beginning and end of
your session.

- Practise this technique until:
  - You feel that your sleep is OK.
  - Somebody else confirms the changes.
  - You are able to keep your mouth taped quite
    comfortably all night.
  - You no longer need the CPAP.

If, having tried all the techniques above, you still cannot
let the CPAP go, you should consider enrolling in a Breath
Connection workshop. It is possible that your condition is
quite serious, or that you did not practise the exercises
correctly, or that an associated disease plays a major role in
your sleep problem and some extra measures need to be
taken.

If you are successful in ridding yourself of the CPAP
machine, simply continue with the routine for Day 1.

Maximal Pause (MP)

Maximal pause is a powerful way to boost CO_2, improve
blood circulation (especially to the brain), increase O_2 and
stop hyperventilation. Many patients will not need this
measure and will find that ordinary Gentle and Shallow
Breathing exercises described on pages 40-42 will be
enough to solve their snoring and sleep apnoea problems.
However, for some chronic sufferers maximal pause gives

the extra boost they need.

- Start as for Control Pause (see pages 7-8) – no deep breath in or out.
- When you feel you need to take a breath, try to suppress it and keep going for another 5 seconds.
- Follow this with 5 minutes of Gentle Breathing.

Note: It will be more difficult to achieve Gentle Breathing – be prepared to make an effort to get it right.

Maximal pause is a very effective exercise and should be used only as prescribed in the treatment plan above. Unlike CP, which can even be used hourly, MP must be limited.

Warning Signs of Sleep Apnoea

- Snoring (especially loud with periodic cessations).
- Restless sleep with frequent awakenings and a pumping heart.
- Waking up in the night gasping for breath.
- 'Heavy' dreams or nightmares.
- Needing to drink water during the night and waking up with a dry mouth in the morning.
- Bedwetting (in children).
- Breathing problems such as shortness of breath.
- Drowsiness during the day.
- Headaches on waking up in the morning.

Central Apnoea

Central apnoea, or Undine Syndrome, is a serious disorder

in which, due to some organic changes of the central nervous system, the body's automatic breathing rhythm is broken, with the result that sufferers must remember to breathe all the time. It is named after Undine, a woman whose promiscuous husband, according to legend, was deprived of all automatic functions and was able to breathe just as long as he remembered to. Eventually he forgot and died during his sleep.

Sufferers from this complaint should not attempt self-treatment, but should consult a medical adviser or qualified Breath Connection practitioner.

Nightmares

It is estimated that we dream for about a quarter of the time we are asleep. Scientists do not know why we dream, but it is thought that the dream period is necessary to sort out the day's events. Most people remember the last dream before they wake up, although some people never seem to remember their dreams (see page 15).

Nightmares are a different story, as they can be quite disturbing. They may be occasional, due to illness or medication, or they might be more persistent or 'chronic'.

It is interesting to note the connections drawn by researchers over the years between nightmares and breathing. As early as 1891, E. Clodd wrote in *Myths and Dreams* of 'the intensified form of dreaming called nightmare, when hideous spectres sit upon the breast, stopping breath and paralysing motion.' E. Jones wrote in *On the Nightmare* that the 'cardinal features of the malady [are a] sense of oppression or weight at the chest which alarmingly interferes with respiration.'

Jones also quotes letters between two doctors, Bond and Radestock. The former wrote 'I have slept in a chair all night, rather than give the enemy an opportunity of attacking me in an horizontal position'. And the latter explained 'If this interference with breathing increases to the point of suffocation, felt in the waking state as a great difficulty in drawing breath, then there comes about the greatly dreaded nightmare.'

Mountaineers often talk of 'nightmares' they have had in an awakened state: deprived of oxygen at great heights, the brain behaves as though it is on a drug-induced trip. Similarly, acute hyperventilation (see page 6) can trigger a nightmare – a type of panic attack in our dream – and the nervous system and the brain concoct a short 'horror movie' to wake us up.

If you suffer from nightmares check your CP before going to bed, and then again on waking from a nightmare. A dramatic drop in your CP will tell you that hyperventilation is the cause of the problem, so before you do anything else, simply lie down and relax, trying to think about nothing but your breathing.

If your breathing is significantly deeper than when you were upright it may be that being in a horizontal position is causing you to hyperventilate – no wonder that after a few hours of sleep you develop nightmares. If, on the other hand, your breathing does not increase significantly after 10-15 minutes, try thinking about some unpleasant work or duty you have to do. If your breathing increases now it means that your nervous system is quite sensitive and that your thoughts, emotions and memories trigger the nightmares. If neither of these scenarios applies, then over-eating, medication, illness, lack of fresh air or another unknown trigger factor may be responsible.

Of course, it is possible that your problem stems from a combination of any or all of the above, but whatever the trigger factors, hyperventilation is still likely to be at the root of the problem. That being the case you should try the following treatment plan for a full month:

Days 1-3
Practise the following three times a day (before breakfast, lunch or dinner and bed):

CP + GB (5 mins) + CP + SB (5 mins) + CP + SBLA (5 mins) + CP + SB (5 mins) + CP + GB (5 mins) + CP

Days 4-10
Practise the following three times a day:

CP + GB (5 mins) + MP + SB (5 mins) + CP + SB (5 mins) + MP + SB (5 mins) + CP + SB (5 mins) + MP + GB (5 mins) + CP

Days 11-14
Rest. Do not practise breathing techniques at all.

Days 15-18
Repeat routine for Days 1-3.

Days 19-26
Repeat Days 4-10.

Days 27-30
Rest.

Continue with this treatment plan until the nightmares stop and do not recur during 'rest' days. Remember also the golden rules:

- Breathe through your nose at all times.
- Go to bed only when you are sleepy.
- Sleep on your left side or your front in an airy, rather cool room.
- Tape your mouth when you go to bed.
- Resist the temptation to eat a big dinner, and avoid black tea, coffee, alcohol and smoking for 2-3 hours before going to bed.

CASE HISTORY

Lena, a 40-year-old book-keeper, was almost killed in a car accident, as a result of which she had been taking a cocktail of drugs for several months. She suffered from nightmares, often felt that she 'jumped' in the night, and would wake up with a headache in the morning. Lena felt that her mouth was open during the night and, having treated her daughter's asthma through Breath Control, she decided to try it herself. She taped her mouth, tried to sleep on her left side (in spite of having been told by doctors to sleep on her back) and on the very first night had no nightmares. She still woke up with a headache, but persevered. She stopped taking anti-depressants and sleeping pills, and now uses painkillers only occasionally. She firmly believes that taping her mouth and changing her sleeping position saved her mind, if not her life.

Night Terrors

Night terrors differ from nightmares in that they can happen during slow-wave, dreamless sleep. Sufferers may jump out of bed screaming, in a cold sweat, seized by a sudden and unexplained terror. The heart races, the eyes widen, and both mind and body are overwhelmed by fear. It is known that this condition may be exacerbated by sleep apnoea and/or stress, and as such can be easily treated by Breath Connection. Practise the following exercise before breakfast, dinner and bed:

CP + SB (5 mins) + MP + SB (5 mins) + CP + SB (5 mins) + MP + SB (5 mins) + CP

Teeth-Grinding

Tooth-grinding is a common problem experienced by most people occasionally, and some more regularly.

- 85-90 per cent of people sometimes grind their teeth in their sleep.
- For 5 per cent of tooth-grinders the problem is a chronic one.

Research at the Mayo Clinic in the USA has shown that antidepressants can cause tooth-grinding, jaw-clenching and even broken teeth. The most common remedy prescribed for tooth-grinding is a mouth guard to be worn at night. However, this may not be necessary if the mouth is taped at night – a measure that Breath Connection advocates in any case (see page 49).

Sleepwalking

Relatively little is known about sleepwalking, although there are definite links between the frequency of sleepwalking and increased levels of stress, anxiety and tiredness – all of which are, of course, synonymous with hyperventilation. Practising Shallow Breathing during the daytime should, therefore, help to combat sleepwalking at night.

It is also thought that sleepwalking in children may be induced by anxiety about bedwetting. In this case the technique for preventing bedwetting described on page 77 may be helpful for some children.

CHAPTER 5

Children and Sleep

- Surveys show that approximately 20-25 per cent of children between the ages of one and five develop some form of sleep problem.
- According to expert sleep researcher Dr M. Weissbluth of the Chicago Sleep Disorders Center, the sleep problems of over 80 per cent of children do not resolve themselves spontaneously.
- 10-15 per cent of children aged between five and 12 experience at least one episode of sleepwalking.

Every parent wants his or her child to go to bed by themselves and sleep through the night. The reality, however, is that for over 30 per cent of today's parents, this does not seem to happen. Many babies and young children wake up at least once during the night, or they resist going to bed in the first place. Some children suffer from nightmares or have sleepwalking episodes, eventually finding their way into their parent's bed.

With children, although things are much simpler on one level, they are often more complex on another. And there is no real answer to the question how much sleep do children need?

Early Signs of Chronic Problems

If you are lucky enough to catch the earliest signs of a chronic problem in your child – the first asthmatic wheeze or symptoms of eczema, hyperactivity, nightmares, bronchitis, etc. – I would recommend you quickly contact a Breath Connection practitioner, even before going to the doctor. There are two reasons for this. First, the tendency of most doctors to put everybody on symptomatic medication, and even overreacting to the first symptoms and prescribing full-blown asthma medication for a wheeze or cough. And second, the fact that many problems can be fixed just by correct breathing. This is much easier with the first signs of disease than it is with a chronic condition.

Various cough syrups and cold and flu treatments can help the occasional problem, but if you notice that your child is prone to frequent colds or flu, or that the cough or wheeze does not disappear after three or four days, do not persist with a symptomatic treatment that masks the real underlying problem.

Often mood swings, irritability or aggression are taken as classic signs of insufficient sleep. However, these may be symptoms of hyperactivity for example, which no amount of extra sleep will cure. Likewise, parents feel that if it is difficult to wake a child in the morning, he must need more sleep. However the child might simply be in the deep sleep stage (see pages 12-13), when a half an hour later or earlier they would wake up more readily.

As explained earlier, in an ideal world we would not force ourselves into a timetabled way of life, sleeping and eating by the clock. We *should* all eat when we are hungry and sleep when we are tired, yet few of us actually do so, and most of us end up forcing a lifetime's bad habit on our children.

So, although the best advice to parents regarding their children's sleep should be to let them sleep whenever they want to so that they go to bed when they feel sleepy and are left there until they wake up on their own, as most of us know, this really is not the most practical advice to follow.

Children have to get up for school, and have to remain awake during lessons and so on. Individual sleep requirements are no more catered for in a child's world than they are in an adult's. Sadly, however, it may be here that sleep problems begin.

Having said all that, there are ways in which we can improve children's sleep patterns, some of which involve breath control, others which involve nothing more than common sense, determination and consistency on the part of parents.

But before we go any further, let's take a look at what we might expect the average child's sleep pattern to be from birth up to five years of age.

Up to 1 month
New babies tend to fall asleep shortly after a feed, waking up every three hours or so to be fed again. They do not yet differentiate between day and night.

From 1 to 4 months
They are beginning to make a distinction between day and night, waking up more frequently during the day than at night.

At 4 months
At this stage they sleep mainly at night, falling asleep after the evening feed, and possibly sleeping through until early morning. There may only be two daytime sleeps now, probably one in the morning and one in the afternoon.

At 10 months
Babies of this age usually go straight to sleep after their evening feed, but may start to develop a ritual of experimental crying to see how easily they can lure their parents' back! Parents need to assess whether or not there is a genuine problem, which can be anything from a dirty nappy to feeling unwell. If there is no such problem, it is best for parents not to indulge this behaviour as it can quickly become a habit. Most babies are sleeping through the night at this stage.

Between 1 year and 18 months
Most children drop one of their daytime sleeps during this period, replacing it with one longer sleep, often after lunch.

At around age 2
Children of this age may start to go to bed slightly later in the evening. Also at this age they are less likely to need your input in the morning, and are better equipped to play contentedly on their own if they wake up early.

At 2 years
At this age most children are unhappy about taking a daytime nap which means that bedtime in the evening may well be earlier. There is often an extended bedtime routine with children reluctant to let their parents leave.

At 3 years
The bedtime routine should be more relaxed now, although nocturnal anxieties and nightmares can be a common occurrence. There may also be more frequent awakenings in children who are no longer wearing nappies at night.

At 5 years
Children who are now at school all day have a full and demanding schedule, so that most are ready for bed by around 7 p.m. Nocturnal anxiety and nightmares are said to reach a peak at this age.

As a general rule, about once a month parents should check their child's sleep patterns two or three times in the course of a night. If you notice that your child . . .

- Sleeps with his/her mouth open
- Sleeps noisily
- Tosses and turns, and/or
- Sleeps on his/her back

you should act in order to prevent any potential sleep or

BACK OR SIDE?

There are different schools of thought as to how a baby should sleep, i.e. in which position. Current thinking in the UK favours babies sleeping on their backs. However, in the Middle East babies are put to sleep either on their left side or on their fronts. Some people even bind the baby's abdomen in order to prevent hyperventilation.

---

general health problems developing.

For children who are aged from 5-15 years, the following exercise can be used to combat nightmares, snoring, bedwetting and a range of other problems connected with hyperventilation. (If your nose is blocked, breathe out, hold your breath and walk for as long as you can before starting Gentle Breathing. Your nose will unblock.)

- Practise Gentle Breathing (GB) for 2-3 minutes.
- Walk slowly for 1-2 minutes, trying to breathe normally, at if you were at rest.
- Practise GB for 2-3 minutes.
- Walk more quickly for 1-2 minutes, again trying to breathe as if you were at rest, gently and shallowly.
- Practise GB for 2–3 minutes.
- Close one nostril with your finger and walk slowly for 1–2 minutes, breathing gently and shallowly.
- Practise GB for 2-3 minutes.
- Do the same walk with the other nostril closed.
- Practise GB for 2-3 minutes.
- Close the first nostril again and walk quickly for 1–2 minutes.
- Practise GB for 2-3 minutes.
- Repeat the faster walk but this time with the other nostril closed.
- Practise GB for 3-4 minutes.

The child should practise this technique three times a day, before breakfast, dinner and bed. From 7-10 days should be enough to show a considerable improvement in sleep. If there is no improvement after 2 weeks, stop

practising and consult a Breath Connection practitioner –
perhaps you are doing the exercise incorrectly.

If the exercise helped, but did not solve the problem
completely within 4 weeks, you should consult a Breath
Connection practitioner – he may make some adjustments
to the technique, taking into account the child's age and
lifestyle, the seriousness of the problem and so on.

If it solved the problem completely within 4 weeks,
keep practising every day for another 3-4 weeks; then
every second day for 3-4 weeks; then twice a week for 3-4
weeks; then once a week for the next 6 months.

THE GOD OF DREAMS

According to Dutch legend, Ole Lukøe, the god of dreams,
would sit on children's beds as they were going to sleep. He
had two umbrellas, one plain and one with beautiful pictures
painted on it. If a child had been good Ole Lukøe would
open the beautiful umbrella over him, and the child would
dream wonderful fairy tales all night. However, a child who
had been naughty would get the plain umbrella and would
wake up in the morning having seen nothing at all.

'Sleeping Through'

As we saw earlier in the book, nobody sleeps through the
night uninterrupted, without awakenings. From the day
we are born, and throughout our lives, we all go through
different stages of light and deep sleep, as well as normal
cycles of wakening (see page 29). These periods are so brief
that we learn to fall asleep again on our own, and in the
morning we don't even remember having woken at all.

However, for babies and children it is often more difficult to fall asleep again without some form of comforting or intervention from parents.

At first, newborn babies cannot differentiate between night and day. Their stomachs can only hold enough food to last them between three and five hours, at which point they wake up to be fed, and it would be unreasonable for us to expect otherwise. As they grow older their systems mature and they sleep longer at night than during the day. Parents can encourage this by following these guidelines:

- Always try to 'put your baby down' awake, so that they

REWARDS AND CHARTS

A very useful technique in helping to motivate your child is to use a reward system. If they know they will earn a star or a sticker if they manage not to get up during the night, your efforts are more likely to succeed. You might also suggest a small prize, perhaps for winning a star for five consecutive nights. If you do decide to use this incentive scheme, it is important that stars, stickers or prizes are awarded as soon as you get up in the morning so that your child sees a very clear association between 'sleeping through' and receiving their reward.

If you reward your child for good behaviour, helping round the house or whatever, at all costs avoid giving chocolate, nuts or milkshakes because they are all strong allergens and the reward could very easily turn into a punishment. Unfortunately, it is unlikely in our society that you will be able to prevent your child from ever eating these foods, but it is a case of better never than late, and the later the better.

---

don't fall asleep with you and wake up without you. They are much more likely to be contented if they are aware that they are being put to bed.

- Should your baby wake up during the night for a feed or for a nappy change, try not to switch on any lights, and do everything with a minimum of fuss or talking so that the baby is not overstimulated.

- Often babies who have a favourite blanket or toy find it easier to part with their parents at night since they have with them a 'security' object that they associate with sleep.

- A bedtime ritual such as a bath or story is a good idea once the child is slightly older providing a good chance to wind down, as well as creating a sense of familiarity and security.

- Herbal baths can be suitable for babies. Try making a tea using camomile herb and water, then strain it and add it to your baby's bath.

Babies and Sleep

'When I have seen a poor Indian woman in the wilderness, lowering her infant from her breast and pressing its lips together as it falls asleep, fixing its cradle in the open air ... I have said to myself: such a mother deserves to be the nurse of emperors.'

George Catlin, *Notes and Travels Amongst the North-American Indians* (1870)

One of the keys to a good, healthy sleep lies, as we have seen, in breathing through the nose and keeping the mouth shut. George Catlin's comment in the quote above

---

SLEEPING WITH THE MOUTH OPEN

In his book *Notes and Travels Amongst the North-American Indians* (1870), George Catlin wrote as follows on the subject of sleeping with the mouth open:

'I have lived long enough, and observed enough, to become fully convinced of the unnecessary and premature mortality in civilised communities, resulting from the pernicious habit above described; and under the conviction that its most efficient remedy is in the cradle, if I had a million dollars to give, to do the best charity I could with it, I would invest it in four million of these little books and bequeath them to the mothers of the poor, and the rich, of all countries.'

Unfortunately, he could not find a million dollars, and neither did four million copies of his book ever get published, but we would all do well to heed his words and educate our children to breathe correctly from an early age.

---

confirms this, however many parents in the Western world are reluctant to keep an infant's mouth closed by taping it, although it has been proven to be perfectly safe. And of course, it would be difficult to train a baby in breath control techniques. So what course of action remains for the many parents whose babies have sleep problems? The following 'controlled crying' schedule is recommended for babies aged from 3-6 months who will not fall asleep alone, and/or those who have frequent awakenings.

When your baby cries at bedtime or after a night-time awakening, let him cry for five minutes. Then, go into the baby's room and reassure him by talking softly. Then leave the room. Don't pick the baby up. If the crying continues, leave the baby for 10 minutes, then go back into the room, and once again reassure the baby without picking him up. Check the baby again after 15 minutes and continue doing so at 15-minute intervals if the crying has not stopped.

Follow the same routine the next night, only starting with a 10-minute wait, then checking after 15 minutes, and making any subsequent checks after 20 minutes. For each successive night after this add 5 more minutes to each of the first and subsequent checks.

Most babies learn to fall asleep on their own within a week using this method. The key is consistency and determination on the part of the parents. It is a good idea to begin the course over a long weekend if possible, as there will inevitably be a few difficult nights for parents.

A SUMMARY OF THE 'CONTROLLED CRYING' SYSTEM

Night	1st check	2nd check	3rd check	Subsequent checks
1	5 mins	10 mins	15 mins	15 minutes
2	10	15	20	20
3	15	20	25	25
4	20	25	30	30
5	25	30	35	35

And so on.

Sleep Problems in Older Children

Many parents fear that perhaps an underlying problem – whether it's a physical one, hyperactivity, a skin problem that is causing itchiness, feelings of being unloved, anxiety or emotional disturbances (see page 34 for common causes of disturbed nights) – is causing their child to have disturbed nights and this prevents them from taking any firm action. It should be fairly obvious if any of these is the case, and if it is it will probably be difficult for the child to go back to sleep even with intervention. However, if the child is growing and developing well and seems to be happy during the day, it is unlikely that there is any such problem.

So, if you have ruled out other possibilities, and you feel that it is simply a case of your child trying to keep you with him for as long as possible at bedtime or when he wakes up in the night, it is probably time to take the bull by the horns and address the problem. The following tips are designed to help you to prepare yourself:

- Keep a diary of your child's sleep disturbances, and what your responses are.
- Discuss and agree with your partner what changes you would like to make.
- Set yourself small targets to begin with.
- Be consistent; if you feel you are going to 'give in' in the end, then don't try to fight it at the beginning.
- Always back your partner up and be supportive so that what your child sees is a united front.
- Avoid long discussions during the night with your child about why he wakes up.
- Try to give your child as much reassurance and closeness as he needs during the day, so that he does not feel the need for it at night.

On a more practical level, use the following strategies to lay the foundations for a 'good night's sleep':

COMMON CAUSES OF WAKEFULNESS IN BABIES AND YOUNG CHILDREN

• Allergy and hyperactivity. Hyperactive children often have difficulty in sleeping and also tend to be early wakers. Allergy can be a cause of poor sleeping habits (and a contributory factor in hyperactivity too): if your child suffers at all from frequent ear or chest infections, has abnormal thirst and/or poor appetite, eczema or excessive dribbling, it is worth looking into whether an allergy is the cause. (See also allergies, pages 127-128.)

• Colic is widely blamed for sleep problems in babies up to the age of around 3 months, particularly in the evenings.

• Discomfort. A wet or dirty nappy, or feeling too hot or too cold, disturbs some babies much more than others.

• Family atmosphere. Children are very sensitive to their parents' moods and feelings and often respond to any tension by a change in their own behaviour. If you are feeling stressed, your child might react by not sleeping so well.

• Fears and anxieties. Most children have some sort of fear – of the dark, of being alone, etc. – or an anxiety which may be highlighted at night time. These are usually things that you can try to discuss with them, putting their minds at ease.

- Always ensure that your child has had plenty of mental and physical stimulation during the day. Lack of stimulation can play a significant role in a large percentage of children's sleep disorders.

- Establish what you feel to be a reasonable bedtime for your child.

- Develop a bedtime routine to help your child make the transition from day to night in a positive way (a bath, getting into pyjamas, brushing teeth, listening to a

- Headlice and threadworms are notorious causes of sleepless nights. Both cause unpleasant itching and make it difficult for children to sleep.
- Hunger is probably the most common and obvious reason for waking up in small babies, but by 3-4 months your baby should be able to go at least 6 hours without needing a feed.
- Illness – a baby or child who is in pain, or who has a fever will wake more easily than usual. Problems such as these are generally easy to spot and can be dealt with as necessary.
- Sucking – all babies are born with a strong natural urge to suck. Those that find their fingers or thumbs at an early age will be able to satisfy this urge without help from their parents (although thumb-sucking can become problematic when adult teeth are in place). However, if they suck a dummy, they will wake up and cry when they can't find it, and breast fed babies may need their mothers for comfort during the night as well as feeding.
- Teething is blamed for a lot of sleep problems, particularly in babies who are normally good sleepers. Some babies find a little teething gel rubbed into the gums quite soothing, however if frequent awakenings continue over a period of months it is unlikely that teething is the cause.

special story, or simply talking about their day).
- Avoid rough play at this time as this gives out the wrong message.
- Try to make as much of the bedtime ritual as possible take place actually in your child's bedroom.
- Never cancel this special routine as a punishment for bad behaviour earlier in the day.

- Always praise your child in the morning if he has stayed in his bedroom all night.

Bedwetting

Every child is expected to go through a period of bedwetting, but equally, they are all expected to stop at some point. However, in some cases bedwetting continues and can become a problem.

As with most sleep disorders, the precise cause of bedwetting is unknown. It appears that bladder size is not a factor, and neither is the depth of sleep. There is some evidence to suggest that bedwetting is caused by a deficiency of an antidiuretic hormone which is responsible for concentrating the urine in order to decrease its volume and give us a stretch of uninterrupted sleep. With bedwetting children, this hormone does not increase during sleep and they therefore produce more urine than their bladders can hold.

There is a man-made version of the hormone that has been shown to prevent bedwetting, but children who have used it have reported side effects. They have included headaches, dizziness, pain and a runny nose. Other conventional treatments may involve 'moisture alarms', 'night lifting' (which means waking your child periodically through the night), bladder control exercises and habit changing. More successful and certainly less traumatic than any of the above is the Breath Connection solution:

Bedwetting Treatment Plan (for Children Aged 5-15)

- Practise Gentle Breathing (see pages 40-41). (An adult

should place a finger under the child's nose from time to time to check for reduction of air flow.)

- In between Gentle Breathing sessions your child should practise walking slowly at first, then faster, then running around the room with the mouth shut for 3-4 minutes.

To simplify, the programme should work thus:

GB (2-3 mins) + slow walk + GB (3-4 mins) + fast walk + GB (3-4 mins) + run + GB (3-4 mins)

- Repeat three times daily (before breakfast, dinner and sleep).

If after 2-3 weeks the problem has not improved you should consult a breath control practitioner for further advice.

Nightmares and Night Terrors

Children, like adults, experience frightening dreams that can cause them to wake up scared. While no one really knows what causes nightmares, most experts believe that scary dreams develop as children and youngsters attempt to resolve the internal conflicts and inner fears that are a part of normal child development. It is also thought that scary movies or frightening real-life events can play a part in causing nightmares.

Nightmares generally occur in the second half of the night when dreaming is most intense. When a child awakes from a nightmare, physical contact, reassurance and comfort are essential. In the case of night terrors, however (see page 70), parents should try to resist the temptation to comfort or hold their child while the terror is in full flow. Instead, they should watch to make sure that their child is safe from falling out of bed or getting hurt in any way, and remain close by until normal sleep resumes. It is important to warn grandparents or babysitters if a child is prone to night terrors so that they know how to deal with it if necessary.

As we saw in Chapter 4 there are links between nightmares/night terrors and breathing/hyperventilation. If your child does suffer from nightmares, hyperventilation may well be at the root of the problem, and a programme similar to that recommended to adults (see page 39) could be the perfect solution. Consult a qualified breath control practitioner for a plan that takes into consideration your child's age and any other relevant factors, and also follow the tips given (see pages 83-85) which should help to promote a good night's sleep.

Sleep in Adolescents

In a recent survey in the USA, adolescents and young adults (that is between the ages of 12 and 25) were identified as a high-risk group for 'problem sleepiness' – that is daytime drowsiness. In fact it has been found that young drivers (aged 25 or under) are involved in more than one half of car accidents caused by falling asleep at the wheel in the USA.

Many young people today go clubbing into the early hours of the morning and try to compensate by catnapping during the day. In addition to this, alcohol and other stimulants play havoc with their bodies, affecting sleep as well as other functions.

It is unlikely that the average rebellious adolescent will keep to sensible bedtimes and regular hours, and in any case, regularity is not necessarily a key player in achieving quality sleep, as discussed earlier. However, there are a number of recommendations that young people might keep in mind with a view to maximising sleep quality, and minimising daytime drowsiness and other related problems:

- Get into bright light as soon as possible after waking up in the morning, but try to avoid it before bedtime. Light acts as a signal to the brain that it is time to wake up, and the onset of darkness indicates it is time to prepare for sleep.
- Encourage them to get to grips with their internal clock, or circadian rhythm (see page 123). If they can manage to do this they will be able to get maximum benefit from their 'peak' times, when they feel fresh and fully functional, in order to compensate for their 'slump' times – those times when they feel drowsy and unable to perform. It also means that they will know when not to take on activities such as driving, in the knowledge that they are not likely to be at their most alert.
- Avoid stimulants such as coffee, colas and nicotine from lunchtime onwards. Also avoid alcohol as this can have a disruptive effect on sleep.
- Avoid heavy reading, studying, and computer games within one hour of going to bed.

Although the typical adolescent's anti-social sleep patterns can often be inconvenient for the rest of the family and irritating to say the least, they are not generally harmful. If, on the other hand, your adolescent child is sleeping significantly less than usual it might be wise to consider possible causes such as substance abuse, emotional problems, or eating disorders such as anorexia, a well-known sleep inhibitor. Talking and/or counselling are essential in all these cases, and the problem should not be neglected.

Early Warning Signs of Sleep Apnoea in Children

Sleep apnoea is a serious problem and symptoms should not be ignored (see page 65 for more details). Watch your child for early indications of sleep apnoea as follows:

- Does your child snore?
- Does your child have a bedwetting problem?
- Is he restless during sleep, frequently changing position?
- Does he breathe through the mouth and is his/her mouth dry in the morning?
- Is he sleepy or hyperactive during the day?

If your answer is 'yes' to any or all of the above you should take this as a strong signal that treatment is needed to prevent the problem from worsening, and consult a Breath Connection practitioner as soon as possible.

Conventional treatment for sleep apnoea in children is the same as for adults – using a CPAP machine (see pages 58-60). The problems with this treatment are:

- It is effectively a life sentence, because the treatment never ends. The child will grow into an adult who is unable to sleep without artificial ventilation.
- While it may help initially, like many drugs, in the long term it will make the problem worse instead of better because it treats only the symptoms. The underlying disease remains untreated and – like any untreated disease – it will get worse.
- Most importantly, it will increase the child's hyperventilation and create lots of other related health problems.

Breath Connection, on the other hand, addresses the cause of the apnoea, produces a rapid improvement and at the same time helps alleviate all sorts of other problems. It is safe, effective, drug-free and physiologically sound.

SIMPLE TIPS FOR A MORE PEACEFUL NIGHT

- Resist the temptation to be overprotective – don't keep your children's windows shut, or cover the bed too heavily with blankets and duvets. Overheating and a lack of fresh air can induce hyperventilation and should be avoided at all costs.
- If your child has kicked off his blankets or duvet, leave him – trust your child's instincts and do not try to replace the covers.
- Encourage your child to sleep on the front or side.
- Tape your child's mouth if it is open at night.

CHAPTER 6

Sleep and Lifestyle

While snoring, nightmares or illness (see Chapters 4 and 8) all take their toll on the quality of our sleep, there are many less obvious day-to-day factors that can influence it, too. Given that sleep is an integral part of our life as a whole, no sleep solution can be effective if the time we spend awake is not taken into account too. When trying to address sleep problems, general lifestyle has to be a major consideration – if we neglect our waking time, our sleep will suffer. Small changes in the way we eat, exercise or manage stress, for example, could have a positive effect on the way we sleep. We need to ensure that we do not fill all our waking hours with work to the exclusion of outside interests, other forms of mental stimulation, time spent with the family, and so on. This chapter will look at general lifestyle concerns, and ways in which sleep can be improved by addressing them.

Diet

In an ideal world, we would all eat (and sleep) as and when we feel the need to do so (see also Chapter 2), rather than trying to force our bodies to fit in with some sort of socially acceptable timetable. However, for as long as the majority of people continue to schedule meals the rest of us are more or less forced to join them.

Our pattern of eating is important because it can affect sleep through arousal which counters the body's natural urge toward relaxation. Eating a large meal within an hour of bedtime, for example, might make you feel sleepy, but in fact it can increase your metabolic rate and body temperature at a time when they should be decreasing, so making it more difficult to fall asleep.

Weight-loss diets can also contribute toward poor sleep. Very low-calorie diets in particular are problematic, often leading to low energy levels, nutritional deficiency, and hunger, all of which can affect sleep.

Being overweight, on the other hand, can also cause sleep problems. Obesity increases the likelihood of breathing problems such as snoring and sleep apnoea (see pages 54-65). Carrying excessive weight can also encourage arthritic changes in the joints causing pain, which in its turn can disrupt sleep too.

While outright clinical malnutrition is rare in the West these days (with the exception of anorexia nervosa), there is an alarmingly high incidence of 'subclinical' mal-nutrition – a lack of essential nutrients which would not be enough to cause diseases such as scurvy, but which can seriously affect the body's working mechanism, and again, this invariably leads to a disturbance of sleep.

Consider the following when choosing when and what to eat in order to improve your sleep:

- When do you generally eat your largest meal? Try to ensure that it is earlier in the day rather than later – at lunchtime rather than in the evening, for example.

- Eat plenty of fresh fruit and salads, dried fruits, green and root vegetables (these are thought to have a more sedative effect than those growing above ground), whole grains, pulses, fish and free-range chicken (in preference to red meats); eat a moderate amount of fats, eggs, cheese and other dairy products.
- Eat protein-rich foods earlier in the day, and unrefined carbohydrates such as potatoes, pasta and rice later on as they are said to have more of a sedative effect. There is research to suggest that certain foods, when combined with carbohydrates, lead to the production of tryptophan, an amino acid that acts as a building block for serotonin (see page 18). These foods include milk, eggs, meat, nuts, fish, hard cheeses, bananas and pulses.
- If you really do need to lose weight, try to do so by lifestyle management involving a good diet and moderate exercise, rather than undertaking extreme low-calorie diets.

Apart from the two cardinal rules, namely eat only when you are hungry and do not overeat, there are a few basic guidelines that are worth following:

- Eat fresh, whole, unprocessed foods wherever possible, avoiding chemical additives and preservatives.
- Eat plant-based foods such as vegetables and grains.
- Avoid junk food and fried foods.
- Reduce your intake of high-protein foods such as meat, fish, nuts and seafood. These increase hyperventilation and can therefore affect how you sleep.

- Avoid chocolate and milk.
- Use sea salt (which is now commonly available) rather than table salt.
- Try to chew your food for longer – a principle also recommended by yoga practitioners.

FOODS TO AVOID TO HELP IMPROVE SLEEP

The following foods should be avoided as far as possible:

- Foods that give you heartburn, as well as fatty or greasy foods, within two hours of bedtime.
- Refined carbohydrates (white flour and sugar) which fill you up but don't give you any real fuel.
- Processed foods containing any chemical additives. In particular tartrazine and monosodium glutamate can disrupt sleep patterns.
- Excess salt.
- Caffeine in tea, coffee, colas and chocolate.

I can't stress enough the importance of giving up the once almost mandatory 'English breakfast'. So many people all over the country used to sit down to high-protein bacon and eggs, toast and marmalade and 'a nice cup of coffee' – probably without even being hungry. This is not a real problem for those who do heavy physical work, as they will produce enough carbon dioxide during the day to burn it off. But for the increasing number of us who lead a more sedentary lifestyle, for example sitting in front of a computer screen all day, it is totally inappropriate to eat as if there were no tomorrow and start the day by ruining our breathing and health. It is no problem, of course, to have breakfast first thing in the morning if you are hungry, but try to make it something healthier. Whilst everyone would agree that overeating is bad for you, very few realize that overeating doesn't necessarily mean putting an excessive amount of food in the stomach. A little food eaten at the wrong time – when you are not hungry – is still overeating.

Research shows that in some 80 per cent of people who complain of feelings of tiredness all the time, the problem lies not with their sleep, but in nutritional deficiencies which can be dealt with easily by improving their diet.

Caffeine and Smoking

Caffeine, in tea as well as in coffee, stimulates the central nervous system and the respiratory system, causes hyperventilation. It also increases urination, and affects the quality of sleep by changing its 'architecture' so that there is less REM sleep (see pages 13-14).

While you need not necessarily cut out tea and coffee altogether, it is a good idea to be aware of their effects and to watch your breathing closely even after just one cup. It is also worth trying to restrict your caffeine intake to the morning hours – some researchers have found a noticeable effect on the heart as much as 10 hours after consumption.

The effects of smoking are well-documented and well-known to most people. While not all smokers feel willing or able to give up their habit altogether, it should be possible for them to keep a close check on their breathing when they smoke and act accordingly. Just as we have seen that changes in breathing may be noted after just one cup of coffee, a cigarette or two can have similar effects. If you can establish a physiologically normal breathing pattern and obtain control over it, you will learn to assess what is good or bad for you and be able to listen to the signals. Just as your breathing gets deeper when you overeat, or eat the wrong foods, perhaps one cigarette does not affect your breathing but a second one might, in which case you should put it out and concentrate on your breathing until it is shallow again.

If you are trying to give up smoking altogether you should be aware of the fact that hyperventilation may develop or worsen as a result of the inevitable stress factor involved. It is not uncommon for asthmatics, and those who suffer from emphysema or heart disease, to find that their conditions worsen after they give up smoking. In order to give up smoking in the safest possible way, try the following:

Day 1
- Try to smoke only when you really feel you want to and not through force of habit.
- Try to draw only three puffs on a cigarette, then put it out; you will probably find that this is enough to satisfy your immediate 'need'.
- Keep count of the number of cigarettes you smoke.
- Draw only one puff on your last cigarette of the day.

Day 2
- Practise the following whenever you feel a craving:

MP + SB (3-4 mins)

If this does not squash the craving, take three puffs of a cigarette.

- When you do smoke, think only of smoking.
- Again, keep count of the number of cigarettes you smoke – you will see that you 'need' fewer.

Day 3
- As for Day 2, smoke on a 'need-only' basis and try to kill the craving with MP and Shallow Breathing.

Day 4
- Practise MP + SB (3-4 mins) whenever you think about cigarettes, or when you see somebody smoking.

Day 5 onward
Continue as for Day 4 until you have not smoked for three days. Once you have managed this you may allow yourself to think about or smell cigaretttes, but continue to concentrate on Shallow Breathing (without MP). You will find that you are able to do this now, and you may even find the smell of cigarettes unpleasant.

THE POWER OF CAFFEINE

Caffeine is used worldwide to accelerate physical and mental activity. Just one cup of coffee contains 100 mg of caffeine; a cup of tea contains 75-100 mg, as does a glass of cola. There is also caffeine in most headache pills.

Alcohol

Some people find that alcohol helps them to fall asleep, as might a big meal (even at lunchtime). This may well be the case, but falling asleep is one thing, and a good, refreshing deep sleep is quite another.

Alcohol relaxes the muscles and in the short term it also makes breathing shallower, but once you are asleep, your body, and in particular your liver is working hard trying to neutralise the alcohol. The effect of the alcohol is to reduce REM sleep (see pages 13-14) in the first phase of sleep, and increase it in the second, so that sleep is shallow with frequent awakenings. After a couple of hours of this, light sleep conditions are perfect for hyperventilation, snoring and heavy dreams. Research has also drawn links between alcohol and sleep apnoea, sleepwalking, bedwetting and nightmares.

A drunken sleep may be a long one, but it is also 'poisonous', causing you to wake up with a heavy head or a full-blown headache, mucus, red eyes and in an irritable mood. So, if you do choose to drink, you should resist the temptation to go to sleep until the effects of the alcohol start to wear off.

Medication

There are various forms of medication that can affect sleep, and many of them create something of a self-perpetuating situation. It is known that sleep problems may be triggered or exacerbated by, among other things, asthma, high blood pressure and depression, and yet the very drugs used to treat these disorders can cause difficulty in sleeping. Breath Connection techniques should always, therefore, be considered first as a way of treating both the primary and the secondary problem (see Chapter 8).

Drugs which can have an adverse effect on sleep include:

- Analgesics containing caffeine.
- Steroids.
- Beta-blockers and some other drugs commonly used to treat high blood pressure.
- Nasal decongestants containing stimulants.
- Many of the drugs used to treat asthma.
- Thyroxin.
- Some anti-depressants.

Exercise and Sport

Yoga, meditation and relaxation exercises can all be very helpful on one level, but depending on how they are practised, they may have a harmful effect on our sleep.

Take meditation for example. If practised correctly it will cause breathing to become very shallow, however some teachers or manuals recommend deep breathing which, as we have seen, causes all sorts of problems. And the same can apply to yoga or to any technique in which the emphasis is on controlled breathing.

To keep ourselves healthy and our bodies in good working order, we must work our muscles as much and as often as possible. Lack of movement (hypokinesia) makes it difficult for the body to free itself of toxins and impairs its ability to function well – rather like filling a car with dirty petrol. Even perfectly fit sportsmen and athletes will start to get sick without exercise – heart rhythms change, the liver function is affected and the body's systems start to deviate from their normal physiological range.

One of the knock-on effects of all these changes is that hyperventilation is induced, and while the overall length of sleep may increase, its quality will suffer so that we see more dreams, wake up more frequently and feel less refreshed.

It is clear, therefore, that for our general well-being, and of course, a good night's sleep, we all need to exercise daily. Having said that, there is no point in exercising or playing sport if you do not control your breathing. When practising any sport you should train yourself to breathe through the nose, and always practise 5-10 minutes of Shallow Breathing at the end of a session.

Note: If you find that you are unable to maintain nasal breathing when playing, or if you have to use medication in order to play (for asthma or blood pressure, for example) you should not be practising the sport in question.

Walking Your Way to Breath Control

To appreciate fully and to master the principles of Breath Connection during movement you should start with walking: breathe through your nose (not deeply) as you walk and gradually increase your pace. After some practice you will find that you are able to jog, run, swim and play tennis or any other sport without deep breathing and with your mouth closed. This sort of breath control will give you increased stamina, but it does take practice.

Breathing Disorders and Exercise

Even people who are chronically ill, for example asthma or emphysema sufferers, should undertake some form of regular exercise. It might be an idea to stick to solo sports (jogging, swimming or cycling) however, until you have really mastered Breath Connection during sport/exercise, so that you can slow down or speed up as and when you want to, rather than having to work at somebody else's pace and disturb your breathing pattern. Follow this routine:

- Check your CP.
- Practise Gentle Breathing for a few minutes, then stand up slowly so as not to disrupt your breathing pattern, and continue with GB for 1-2 minutes in a standing position.
- Start moving – again, very slowly – gradually picking up speed until you feel unable to maintain GB.
- Stop and sit down.

How far you have got by this stage will depend largely on your initial CP, but you will find that you cover more ground with practice.

Note: If/when you develop wheezing or shortness of breath, or you start to cough, you should slow down or stop and get your breath back by practising Shallow Breathing until the wheezing stops. If this does not work, take a puff of your bronchodilator. You may then continue exercising, keeping a careful check on your breathing.

Always check your CP immediately before exercising/ playing sport and again 10-15 minutes afterwards. If it goes down it is an indication that all is not well, and your sleep may suffer as a result. To counter this, reduce the intensity of the exercise or sport you are playing and take more frequent breaks in order to keep better control over your breathing.

Melatonin

Melatonin ('the hormone of darkness') is a natural sleeping medicine. It is a hormone made naturally by the body, but it is also available commercially at health stores and pharmacies in many countries, though not in the UK. In countries where it is legal, melatonin is normally recommended to help restore a healthy sleeping cycle, particularly for people experiencing jet lag.

While it is known that melatonin does work, and that it does not seem to cause any side effects, its long-term effects are still not well understood. Some researchers refer to it as a 'wonder' drug and believe it could be used as an anti-cancer and anti-ageing therapy. Others, however, are more sceptical and feel that there is no real evidence to support these theories.

Apart from the general uncertainty surrounding melatonin, there is also a problem when it comes to establishing the correct dosage. And like any drug, 'miracle' or otherwise, an overdose may be dangerous. Fortunately, CO_2 is once again the answer to our problems, since it plays a vital role in regulating the activity of our hormonal system. So, if we are breathing correctly, our body should be producing enough melatonin on its own, and there should be no need for us to supplement it.

Relaxation and Meditation

Normally, the onset of sleep is a drowsy, relaxed state – a sort of peaceful letting go. Ideally, we would all simply drift into sleep when we get into bed, but unfortunately for many of us life in the 21st century is too busy and stressful to allow this to happen easily. Relaxation is an art that many of us have not taken the time to master and learning, or re-learning it, is vital. When we relax, we are better equipped to breathe correctly, and from there the rest is plain sailing.

It is a common misconception that watching television, going to the cinema or a restaurant, and socialising are relaxing pastimes. Of course, they are all important and all serve a purpose, but it would not be correct to say that they are truly relaxing. Real relaxation involves 'switching off' the active right brain, and that part of the nervous system that psyches us up for action. It works against all the negative effects of stress and also helps to strengthen the immune system. There is even some research to suggest that very deep states of relaxation can alter body chemistry to the extent of producing hormones, called endorphins, which can improve mood and relieve pain.

Meditation is known to have similar effects to those of relaxation, although it is geared more towards the mind and spirit than the body. In fact it has also been noted that people who meditate regularly find that they can function well on less sleep, because their systems are fully rested and restored through meditation (see pages 106-108).

Relaxation Techniques

In order to benefit fully from relaxation you need to allow yourself at least twenty minutes daily for getting it right. Learning to 'let go' without fearing a loss of control is vital, and it takes time and dedication to learn this. The following techniques should help you to relax; you might find it beneficial to conjure up some form of pleasing mental imagery, or to play soothing background music as you work on them.

Technique 1
- Sit comfortably with your back supported, your feet flat on the floor, your hands in your lap and your eyes closed.
- Alternately tense and relax all the muscles in your body, working from your head to your toes (or vice versa), including your jaw, and even your tongue. Work very slowly, and concentrate your mind on feelings of heaviness and warmth in your limbs.
- When you have been through your whole body, take a moment to observe whether there are still any tense muscles, and try to relax them.
- Now spend the remaining time simply enjoying the sensation of relaxation. At the end of your session, get up slowly to avoid any feelings of dizziness.

Technique 2
- In a sitting or lying position, stretch your whole body, then relax.
- Sense the waves of relaxation as they spread through your body when you breathe in, and feel the tension

leave your body as you breathe out.

Technique 3
Tiredness and tension in the head area can be particularly problematic. Try the following to release tension in this area:

- Roll your head slowly clockwise and then anti-clockwise, three times each way, allowing it to drop heavily. Allow your jaw to open and your eyes to close.
- Slowly drop your head forward, to each side, then back, as far as possible, stretching the neck muscles as you do so. Repeat 10 times.
- Keeping your head level, turn it from side to side 10 times slowly, then another 10 times more quickly.

Meditation Techniques

As for the relaxation exercises above, you need to set aside time exclusively for meditation when you know you will not be interrupted or distracted. Meditation works by emptying your conscious mind of thoughts, and by directing them away from yourself and your problems. By doing this you are able to transcend ordinary levels of consciousness and open up pathways to unconscious thought and experience. This is greatly beneficial in breathing terms since it causes your breathing to become slower and more shallow.

There is no one correct position in which to practise meditation. Any of the following is acceptable:

- Sitting on a hard chair, your back supported, feet together, and hands resting lightly in your lap.
- Sitting cross-legged on the floor, body upright, arms relaxed, hands resting on your knees.
- The 'lotus' position in which you sit on the floor, with both feet on opposite thighs, hand resting palm-up on your knees.
- Sitting on the floor with your back against a wall, legs outstretched, knees and feet together, and hands resting on your thighs.
- Lying flat on the floor, shoulders and neck relaxed, and hands by your sides.

Once you are in a comfortable position in a quiet, tranquil environment, you are ready to meditate. Here are some techniques:

- Repeat a single word mentally. Focus your attention on this word, and whenever you find your mind wandering, bring it back to your chosen word.
- Try focusing on your breathing, counting each breath going from 1 to 10. Exclude all thoughts from your mind, and try to visualise each number as you count by mentally 'planting' them in the centre of your stomach. Try to let each number melt gently into the next.
- Contemplate an object, such as a perfectly formed flower or symbolic design or flickering candle. As you do so, silently repeat to yourself a single sound.

Note: Ideally, relaxation and meditation exercises should be practised with some sort of professional guidance. However, the above techniques serve as an introduction to these disciplines and should certainly help to pave the way to a highly, satisfying, good night's sleep.

Relationships

In today's hectic world where so many of us are busy trying to juggle our careers, homes and hobbies while worrying about keeping afloat financially, stress is one of the biggest factors we have to deal with. It is also one of the most common causes of sleepless nights, and there is nothing quite like a family or domestic crisis to induce it!

There are all sorts of problems and issues that can lead to quarrels or disputes within relationships, but whatever the cause, the effect will always be the same – hyper-ventilation. Any situation in which you are angry, shouting, arguing, crying or feeling depressed is one in which you hyperventilate. And this compounds an already emotive situation because when you hyperventilate your mind is clouded and unclear; it is working overtime and yet quite unproductive since you are unable to think straight. You feel emotionally and sometimes physically drained, and yet are unable to sleep well.

Understanding the vicious cycle of argument – hyper-ventilation – lack of sleep – irritability – argument, etc., can help to overcome it. It would be unrealistic to suggest that we should never disagree with each other, particularly since in some instances the closer we are to someone the more sensitive certain issues become. However, by learning to control our breathing at all times we may be able to avoid setting off the chain reaction in which hyperventilation is a key link, however hurt or enraged we are feeling (see also stress, pages 146-148).

Travel and Jet Lag

It is considered nothing these days to take several flights in a week, crossing one or more time zones. And yet the reality is that so much travel does take its toll.

When you reach your destination you may already be at a disadvantage. With very little leg room on the flight it is difficult to stretch your legs or to move around at all, your neck and leg muscles may be aching, you may have slept only fitfully and not deeply, and you will be missing the restorative effects of sleep. You may also be experiencing physical symptoms in response to a change in climate, or air-conditioning, and it is often hard to eat breakfast, for example, in what feels like the middle of the night. It takes a while for your body and mind to catch up with one another and to start functioning effectively within a new time zone, and this is the all too common phenomenon known as jet lag – yet another by-product of the frenzied lifestyle that so many of us lead today.

To help you sleep well when you are travelling, try the following:

- When you feel sleepy during a flight practise 10 minutes of Gentle Breathing followed by 10 minutes of Shallow Breathing.
- Try not to eat on the plane, or eat as little as possible. (Those with a low CP – below 15 seconds – should be particularly careful in this respect.)
- Do not smoke or drink alcohol during a flight.
- Get up as frequently as you can without annoying your neighbours (!) to stretch your leg muscles and revive your circulation.

- To restore normal sleeping patterns as soon as possible on arrival use the technique on pages 38-39 to fight drowsiness, or take a short nap (15-20 minutes) if you cannot resist. (See also Melatonin, page 103)

THE PERFECT PILLOW?

There is an old fairy tale that tells of a Tsar who suffered terribly from insomnia. Convinced that his pillow was the root of the problem he assembled the wisest men in his kingdom and asked their advice.

The first wise man proposed a pillow made from the finest Chinese silk. Having already tried this the enraged Tsar called for him to be put to death, and summoned the next man. He, in his turn, suggested that a pillow made from Siberian blue sable would put the Tsar out of his misery, but sadly, he met the same fate.

And so it went on, until at last, one wise old man told him: 'Your majesty, without a doubt, your palm is the best pillow.' The Tsar was incredulous, not knowing if the man was trying to help him or simply ridicule him. But he tried it none the less, and was delighted at the outcome. The strange old man was rewarded generously, and as for the Tsar, he never had another sleepless night.

The truth is, if a person is really tired, they will sleep no matter what pillow they use – even a stone would do. However, if they try to sleep before their body is ready, no pillow will help, whatever the quality.

Air-Conditioning

It is not uncommon these days for people to work or sleep in offices, houses, flats or hotels with the windows firmly shut and an air-conditioning system humming gently in the background. While these systems may be an effective means of cooling the air, at the same time they are stripping it of its negative ions, making it stale, unhealthy to breathe and certainly not conducive to good quality sleep. You might, for example, sleep too long, then still feel tired on waking up, or you might have a fitful night with several awakenings. There really is no substitute for an open window and fresh air when it comes to healthy breathing, and the chance of a good night's sleep.

Seasonal Affective Disorder (SAD)

Just as animals react to the changing seasons with alterations in mood and behaviour, so do we. Most people find that they eat and sleep slightly more in winter than they do the rest of the year, and that they dislike the short days and dark mornings. Some people, however, find that their reaction to the winter months is more severe, causing disruptive symptoms and considerable distress. These people are suffering from seasonal affective disorder (SAD), caused by a lack of bright light in the winter.

Our sleep-wake cycle, or circadian rhythm (see page 123), is the mechanism around which our other bodily rhythms – hormonal, physiological, neurological and behavioural – revolve, and it is the natural light-dark cycle that signals the time of day. When too little natural bright light gets to the brain, or when bright light enters the brain at the 'wrong' time of day, it disrupts the timing of the 'clock' which can then fail to synchronise the body's rhythms. The first indication that this has happened is a disruption in sleep, as well as some or all of the symptoms which are described below.

Unfortunately for shift workers – who tend to see less daylight all year round, but particularly in the winter – they are among those people most likely to experience SAD. Some of the most common symptoms of this syndrome are overeating, depression, irritability, lethargy and lowered resistance, all of which can cause sleep problems. Sufferers often find that they sleep *more* than they would like to, but that their sleep is not refreshing or restorative, and that they have difficulty in getting out of bed. There is also a tendency toward more frequent napping. Practising the Basic Insomnia Course (see pages 43-46) should help, but sufferers may find they have to practise it at unusual times – when other people are asleep.

SUFFERING FROM SAD

- Around 2 per cent of people in northern Europe suffer badly from full-blown SAD, while around 10 per cent complain of milder symptoms ('winter blues').
- The incidence of SAD worldwide increases with distance from the equator, except when there is snow on the ground and it becomes less common.
- More women than men are diagnosed with SAD.

CHAPTER 7

Special Cases: Women, the Elderly and Shift Workers

Women and Sleep

- One in four American women over the age of 65 are reported to suffer with sleep apnoea (see pages 57-65).
- 66 per cent of sufferers of nocturnal eating disorder (see page 143) are thought to be women.
- According to a National Sleep Foundation Gallup poll, taken in 1996, women suffer from more night-time pain in the form of migraine, headache, chronic fatigue syndrome and fibromyalgia than men.
- Almost a third of women report using either caffeine, over-the-counter remedies or prescription drugs to help combat the effects of day-time fatigue.

Certain conditions unique to women, such as the menstrual cycle, pregnancy and menopause, can affect sleep quality largely because of changing levels in hormones, for example oestrogen and progesterone, but also because of associated pain and discomfort. Resulting day-time fatigue can have serious consequences affecting alertness at the wheel, work, or caring for children.

The Menstrual Cycle

Changes in women's bodies (and sometimes mood) occur at different times in the menstrual cycle, and some women complain, for example, that their sleep is disturbed because they feel bloated. The rise in progesterone after ovulation may cause some women to feel tired, but on the whole poor quality sleep is more likely to be at the beginning of the cycle when bleeding starts, with an average of two to three disturbed nights per cycle. It has also been found that as progesterone levels begin to decrease again, some women find difficulty in falling asleep. Symptoms of premenstrual syndrome (PMS) such as headaches, irritability, bloating and abdominal cramps can also contribute to sleep problems.

There are some basic measures that can help to alleviate sleep problems brought on by menstruation:

- Try to take regular exercise but not within three hours of going to bed. Exercise can help to relieve symptoms of PMS, and thus create better conditions for good quality sleep.
- Avoid foods that are high in sugar, salt and caffeine.
- Try to reduce your alcohol intake.

SNORING IN PREGNANCY

A reported 30 per cent of pregnant women snore for the first time during pregnancy because of increased swelling in the nasal passages. In severe cases this can lead to sleep apnoea (see pages 57-65) which disrupts sleep and may also affect the unborn foetus.

Pregnancy

Pregnancy is an exciting, yet physically demanding time for women. Symptoms such as body aches, heartburn, nausea, leg cramps, along with foetal movements and emotional changes which may include depression, anxiety or worry, can all conspire to interfere with sleep.

High levels of progesterone in the first trimester (three months of pregnancy) increase feelings of daytime sleepiness, and there may also be a need for frequent urination during the night, which in turn can add to drowsiness during the day.

During the second trimester progesterone levels are still on the rise, but more steadily now, allowing for better sleep. The foetus moves up, relieving pressure on the bladder, which also increases the likelihood that sleep quality may be better than it was during the first trimester. And it is certainly greatly needed.

The majority of pregnancy-related sleep problems are experienced during the final trimester, when physical discomfort, along with heartburn and leg cramps, reach a peak. The foetus also begins to put pressure on the bladder again, which means more frequent visits to the toilet during the night.

The following tips may help to improve sleep quality during pregnancy:

• Sleeping on the left side is recommended to everyone, at all times (see pages 47-48), but can be particularly beneficial during the third trimester of pregnancy as it allows for a better blood flow to the foetus, and to your uterus and kidneys.

- Avoid spicy and acidic foods to prevent heartburn.
- Try to exercise regularly but sensibly (take professional advice) to improve circulation and reduce leg cramps.
- Eat small, frequent bland snacks (such as crackers) to prevent nausea.

Using Breath Connection Exercises during Pregnancy

For the first six months of pregnancy there is nothing to preclude you from following the normal Breath Connection exercises to combat insomnia or other sleep problems. It is only in the final trimester that exercises should be different:

- Practise Relaxation and Meditation (see pages 104-108) for 30-40 minutes a day for 7-10 days
- Then go 'one step further' by adding underbreathing – deliberately start taking in less air during your meditation sessions. Check your CP before and after to make sure you are achieving the desired result, a normalising of CO_2. *Do not practise* deep breathing techniques as this can decrease the supply of oxygen both to yourself and to your baby – and, of course, make your sleep worse.
- Learn how to walk with good breath control, not breathing deeply. This will be more difficult in the later stages of pregnancy, when you are carrying a lot of extra weight, but you should breathe through your nose with your mouth shut. If you feel the need to open your mouth to breathe, stop to catch your breath instead.
- Understanding nervousness while expecting a baby, especially if it is your first, may make you breathe more and sleep less. Be aware of the first signs of hyper-

ventilation and try to deal with them the moment they appear. Stop what you are doing, sit down, relax and bring your breathing down.

• Avoid overeating which leads to overbreathing.

• Of course, you should avoid caffeine, chocolate and smoking, all of which will affect you more when you are pregnant and are having breathing difficulties.

SLEEP PROBLEMS IN PREGNANCY

According to research carried out in America in 1998:

• On average, women report disturbed sleep for 2-3 days per cycle.

• More women than men are reported to suffer from Restless Leg Syndrome (RLS) (see pages 145-146).

• Up to 15 per cent of pregnant women develop RLS during their third trimester.

• 51 per cent of pregnant women take at least one weekday nap.

• 78 per cent of women report that their sleep is disturbed more during pregnancy than at other times.

Menopause

When a woman approaches the menopause there is a decline in the hormone oestrogen. This can cause hot flushes (unexpected feelings of heat all over the body), sometimes accompanied by sweating, and they can often interfere with sleep. While the overall quantity of sleep may not be affected, there is definitely a drop in quality, and frequent awakenings may also cause day-time fatigue.

SLEEP PROBLEMS DURING THE MENOPAUSE

- Approximately 25 per cent of menopausal women in the USA take some form of hormone replacement therapy.
- 35-40 per cent of menopausal women suffer from sleep problems.
- 36 per cent reported hot flushes during sleep.

Women who experience sleep problems during the menopause should first treat the primary cause – hormonal imbalance, rather than sleep *per se*. The conventional treatment of Hormone Replacement Therapy (HRT) is helpful to many women and is thought to help prevent osteoporosis. However, it may also bring a greater risk of breast cancer and some women experience increased bleeding if they take too much oestrogen. The effectiveness of HRT is also reduced if you are taking antibiotics, or medication for blood pressure problems or epilepsy.

Some women prefer to take complementary medicines such as high doses of soya or red clover (plant-based oestrogen). Again, this is effective for some but not all women.

I would certainly recommend Breath Connection techniques to menopausal women because this is the only currently known treatment which deals directly with normalising the body's levels of carbon dioxide, described by scientist Yandell Henderson, working at Yale University in the early part of the twentieth century, as the 'chief hormone'. Normalising CO_2 will also redress the hormone imbalance, so you will not need to gamble with trying to find the right level of artificial hormones.

The comprehensive treatment of menopausal symptoms with Breath Connection is specific to the individual, and I would recommend that you visit a qualified practitioner, but you can try the following right now:

- Whenever you develop hot flushes, mood swings, etc., or feel that they may be coming on, sit down, relax, breathe out and hold your breath for as long as you can. Then start breathing through your nose, as shallowly as possible.
- Repeat 3-4 times during the next 15-20 minutes and see what happens. You may be feeling much better!
- Practise Shallow Breathing (see pages 41-42) for another 5-10 minutes.
- If you wake up during the night because of pain or hot flushes, sit up and do the same exercise.

You may have to repeat this routine several times during the day, depending on the frequency and severity of your problems. Unfortunately, it can only help the symptoms, it can't prevent them – for that, you need the full course of treatment! But you can get fast relief just through breathing when even powerful drugs can't do much.

Sleep in Old Age

The changes that ageing brings creep up on us slowly, sometimes almost unnoticed. However, sooner or later we all become aware that perhaps our own, or our relatives' eyesight or hearing, for example, is less keen than it once was. Similarly, it is a well-established fact that elderly people sleep less than young people. It's not that our sleep requirements change as we age, it is simply that changes in health, lifestyle and behavioural patterns mean that our bodies do not work in the same way as before. The following are all factors that conspire to make sleep more elusive in old age:

- Chronic pain, osteoporosis, arthritis, breathlessness and constipation.
- Bereavement, loneliness, depression and changes in mental attitude.
- Reduction in, or a lack of physical activity, and/or mental stimulation.
- The accumulative effects of long-term use of alcohol and tobacco.
- A dramatic rise in the incidence of snoring with advancing age, along with its associated problems (see Chapter 4).
- A decrease in the production of melatonin and growth hormone.
- Less exposure to natural light (see also SAD, page 111).
- Dietary changes.
- Changes in the body temperature cycle.
- Medication – older people are much more likely to be taking a variety of medications that may adversely affect their sleep, particularly if they have been taking them long-term.

In addition, recent research suggests that the ageing bladder may contribute to sleep disturbances in the elderly. There is also evidence to suggest that the biological clock (see 'circadian rhythm' on page 123) that regulates our physiological systems begins to run down, so that it drives the sleep-wake cycle less efficiently than before, and is less able to sustain periods of long sleep.

HOW PAIN AFFECTS SLEEP

A 1996 National Sleep Foundation Gallup poll revealed that of night-time pain sufferers:

- 30 per cent experienced arthritis pain at night, the number rising to 60 per cent in those over 50. Sufferers in this age group reported loss of an average of 2.2 hours of sleep approximately one night in three.
- 64 per cent experienced back pain.
- From 44-56 per cent experienced headaches, muscular aches and pain, leg cramps and sinus pain.

Any or all of the above conditions may set in or worsen with advancing age, and these statistics highlight the potential for increased sleep problems in older people.

Sleep Changes in Old Age

As we grow older we might expect the following changes in our sleep:

- **Sleep structure (or stages).** Middle-aged and elderly people (particularly men) tend to spend less time in deeper sleep, while the percentage of REM sleep remains relatively stable. There is also some research to suggest that elderly men have more passive dreams while older women have more active, outgoing dreams.
- **More frequent awakenings.** Because sleep is shallower there is an increased tendency to wake up during the

night, and many elderly people find it difficult to fall back to sleep.

- **Higher incidence of conditions that have an adverse effect on sleep quality and duration.**
- **More frequent naps.** Fragmented night-time sleep causes more daytime sleepiness, and reduced activity provides more opportunity to counter this with catnaps.

Solving Sleep Problems in Old Age

It may appear from the above that sleep problems in old age are a necessary evil. However, it is important to note that there are plenty of elderly individuals who experience few sleep problems, if any at all.

Furthermore, remember that changes in sleep patterns may point to an underlying sleep disorder. For example sleep apnoea (see pages 57-65), restless leg syndrome (see pages 145-146), and periodic leg movement disorder (see page 145) are all more common in old age, and one of these may be at the root of your problem. Depression (see pages 134-136) too can be a factor.

All of the above can be dealt with using breath control techniques, irrespective of age, and a consultation with a qualified breath control practitioner may help to highlight particular areas to work on.

In addition, there are plenty of general measures that should be taken. Older people who are more able should try to keep themselves involved in some sort of physical activity, even if it is just taking a daily walk, since inactivity is a strong predisposing factor in poor sleep. It is also important to keep alert mentally, whether by reading, doing puzzles, crosswords, or attending talks and lectures. Mental stimulation is vital.

Most importantly, it is never too late to try and solve your sleep problems, and there is no reason why older people should simply accept them as a hopeless inevitability. You can never be too old to embark on a breath correction programme. After all, for as long as you are breathing, it is worth learning to breathe correctly.

Working Shifts

Shift workers perform vital tasks whether their work is in hospitals, in the emergency services, the police force, or in travel, transportation or manufacturing industries. However, in most cases, shift workers do not get enough quality sleep. Often it is difficult for them to remain alert at night, yet just as hard to fall asleep and remain asleep during the day, and the sleep that they do get is less restorative than that of night sleepers.

The human body naturally follows a 24-hour period of wakefulness and sleepiness that is regulated by an internal 'circadian' clock. This clock, which we have in common with all other living creatures and plants, is linked to nature's cycle of light and darkness, and helps to regulate body temperature, hormones, heart rate and other functions. The natural urge to sleep in humans is strongest between midnight and 6 a.m. and it is very difficult for us to reset our circadian clock in order to condition it to want to sleep at other times.

The following tips may help shift workers to set the scene for a more restful and restorative sleep:

- Take a warm bath before bed.
- Darken the bedroom.
- Use some sort of 'white noise', such as a fan, to block out other household noises.
- Avoid caffeine within 5 hours of bedtime.
- Avoid the temptation to drink alcohol after work; it may help you to relax and unwind, but it also interferes with sleep, causing disturbances.
- Eat a light snack before going to sleep – don't go to bed too full or too hungry.
- If you do any form of exercise in the workplace, it is extremely important that you do so at least 3 hours before your bedtime since this causes stimulation and raises the body temperature which can interfere with sleep.

Breath Connection Advice for Shift Workers

Shift workers are really suffering from a similar problem to jet lag (see pages 109-111). You break the normal pattern of 'night is for sleeping, day is for activity' and suffer the after effects; you feel sleepy or wakeful at the wrong time. The following tips should help.

- Get rid of the psychological pressure that it is harmful not to sleep at night like 'normal' people, or not to get a 'proper' 8 hours' sleep, or to have your sleep broken. None of these things is harmful; in fact it is quite healthy to sleep a little here and there rather than sleeping solidly for 8 hours or even more. (Can you see a similarity with eating?)
- Of course, the problem is then that you have to work

SHIFT WORKERS AND SLEEP

- More than 22 million Americans work shifts – a number that is growing by 3 per cent each year.
- 10-20 per cent of shift workers report falling asleep on the job, usually during the second half of their shift.
- Shift workers are said to experience more stomach problems (in particular heartburn and indigestion), menstrual irregularities, colds, flu and weight gain than their daytime counterparts.
- There is an increased risk of workplace and road accidents among shift workers, particularly on the journey to and from work.
- Studies show that napping is an effective tool for shift workers who need to maintain a high degree of alertness and attention to detail, and who need to make quick decisions.

---

when you may be really sleepy. In that case, use the energy-giving Maximal Pause (see page 64) which will make you feel more alert. Also, wash your face with cold water. Resist the temptation to drink endless cups of coffee as you will pay a heavy price later for staying awake now. You'll discover this when you need more and more coffee to keep you awake and it then takes longer and longer to fall asleep when you want.

- On the other hand, if you are sleepy and can afford to take a nap, do it. Even a 5-minute nap can make a big difference if you take it at the peak of your sleepiness. You will feel really refreshed. Do this several times in the course of your shift if you have the sort of work that allows it.

- Make sure you have plenty of air in your room – it will improve the quality of your sleep if you do take a nap, and it will help you to stay more alert when you are supposed to be awake. Also make sure the room is not too hot.
- If you can manage 5-6 hours of sleep every day, you should not be worrying about lack of sleep. However psychologically difficult it may feel, from the physiological point of view you are getting enough sleep, or 'core sleep', and your health will not be affected. It may just take you a little time to get used to it.

CHAPTER 8

Conditions Affecting Sleep and How to Deal with Them

Allergies

Allergies are double trouble as far as sleep is concerned. Not only do their symptoms – sneezing, wheezing, a blocked nose, breathing difficulties, itching and an upset stomach – cause sleep problems but their orthodox treatment – antihistamine – often causes drowsiness during the day and insomnia at night.

As we have seen elsewhere, treatment of allergies with drugs addresses not the cause but the symptoms, and is therefore ultimately ineffective. In order to understand why this is, we need to understand what an allergy is.

We know that an allergy is a disease of the immune system, so that the cause lies inside us. An allergic reaction is triggered by a foreign substance – known as the allergen – from which the impaired immune system is unable to protect us. Our immune system is strong when the pH (acid-alkaline) balance lies within physiological norms; however, hyperventilation is known to shift this balance in as little as 1-2 minutes with the result that normal reactions become allergic. It is therefore essential that hyperventilation is dealt with as part of any allergy treatment plan.

The following exercise (be sure that you follow the specified times) should be practised at the first signs of an allergic reaction:

CP + SB (1-2 mins) + CP+5 secs + SB (1-2 mins) + CP+10 secs + SB (5 mins)

Arthritis

Rheumatoid arthritis is thought to be caused by an unspecified (and therefore untreatable) infection, while the cause of osteoarthritis is unknown. Sufferers of both forms of arthritis often experience pain on waking up in the morning and also wake up in pain during the night, which means that their sleep quality is impaired. This can be quite unsettling.

The most effective form of symptomatic relief is known to be steroids. However, we know that hyperventilation suppresses the body's natural production of steroids, which means that by reducing hyperventilation we might not only reduce painful episodes naturally, we may also eliminate the need for prescribed steroids, and with it their side effects. Of course, reducing pain also means improving sleep.

Try the following exercise which is very good at helping to relieve pain from arthritis. (If this does not work, take your medication, then try the exercise again, pre-empting the pain if possible.)

MP + SB (3-4 mins) + MP + SB (3-4 mins) + CP + SB (5-6 mins)

Asthma

Asthma is a condition in which the smooth muscles of the walls of the bronchi (the tubes which conduct air to the lungs) contract in spasm. This causes narrowing of the airway, resulting in shortness of breath and wheezing. In spite of the fact that the asthma trigger-factors are well known (e.g. dust, cold weather, animals, tobacco and sport), its actual cause is unknown. The orthodox medical treatment is therefore symptomatic.

If you are an asthmatic and your condition is waking you up one or more times during the night, the problem is clearly out of control and the following course of action should be taken:

- If you use inhaled steroids you should double your dose.
- If you use oral steroids, take one extra 5mg tablet; chew it and wash it down with warm or hot water for quicker absorption.

As a general rule:

- Establish the correct dose of steroids for you so that:
  - Your asthma does not wake you at night.
  - One 'puff' of a bronchodilator is enough to open up the airway.
  - You are gradually able to stop using long-lasting bronchodilators (within a few days).
  - You only use nebulisers in case of emergency. Switch to inhalers instead.
- Increase your steroids only when your asthma is worse,

and decrease them when it's better.
- Take oral steroids straight away if you get no relief from 1-2 puffs of an inhaler.
- Immediately clamp down on breathing through your mouth, day and night.
- At the first sign of an attack practise Shallow Breathing for 5-6 minutes. If this does not work take one puff of your inhaler.

Once you have made some headway with your symptoms and you feel that your condition is improving, practise the following 3 times a day (i.e. before breakfast, lunch and dinner):

CP + SB (5 mins) + CP + SBLA (5 mins) + CP + SB (5 mins) + CP + SBLA (5 mins) + CP + SB (5 mins) + CP

Blocked Nose

A blocked nose, regardless of its cause, makes us breathe through the mouth, which in turn leads to hyper-ventilation. It is a vicious cycle because the more we breathe through the mouth, the more we hyperventilate, and the more blocked our noses become, and so on. In particular, a blocked nose affects quality of sleep, causing snoring, which contributes to sleep apnoea (see pages 57-65), shallow sleep and, as a result, other sleep problems.

Fortunately, there is a way to unblock the nose without resorting to medication which only offers symptomatic relief, and is therefore useless in the long term. Try the following breathing formula whenever your nose is blocked, but not more than 5-6 times a day.

- Sit down and breathe out. It is important that you feel quite relaxed.
- Remain seated, hold your breath and firmly pinch your nose.
- After a few seconds stand up and, still holding your breath, walk across the room for as long as you can, then sit down again.
- Stop pinching your nose and start breathing gently – not deeply – through your nose. You should soon notice an improvement.

This exercise should keep your nose unblocked for some time. It is generally quite successful. If you find it becomes blocked within minutes of finishing the exercise, you may need further help from a Breath Connection practitioner.

Of course the best cure is to adopt Shallow Breathing as a way of life. Once you develop a new breathing pattern you will beat the problem long term since Shallow Breathing and a blocked nose cannot co-exist. The two are incompatible.

Bronchitis

Inflammation of the bronchi – bronchitis – can be acute or chronic. Either way it causes coughing fits at any time, day or night, and therefore affects quality of sleep. However, while acute bronchitis is caused by bacteria and usually lasts only a few days, the cause of chronic bronchitis is unknown, and the disease can go on for years or even a lifetime.

For either type of bronchitis, it is advisable to try to

stop coughing, regardless of whether the cough is productive (i.e. with mucus) or dry.

Try the following technique whenever you start coughing:

MP + SB (3 mins)

When you feel a coughing fit threatening try:

 CP + SB (3 mins) + GB (5 mins)

Note: If you are in bed always sit up before practising these techniques.

Chronic Fatigue Syndrome

Also known as ME (myalgic encephalitis), chronic fatigue has for some time been the subject of controversy in the medical world: some people believe it is a psychological disorder, others believe its origins to be viral, and another group believes it's an immunological disorder. Whatever its cause, the symptoms include excessive tiredness of which sufferers are acutely aware, and hyperventilation, of which they may or may not be aware. The treatment of chronic fatigue is an extremely delicate process and should be undertaken on a strictly individual basis, under the guidance of a qualified Breath Connection practitioner. Some general principles, however, are as follows:

- Breathe through the nose only.
- Use your bed for sleep only; if you are simply tired and need to rest, do so in a chair.

- Practise the following before breakfast, lunch and dinner:

CP + SB (10 mins) + CP + SB (10 mins) + CP

- Practise the following before bed:

CP + SB (10 mins) + MP + SB (10 mins) + CP

Colds and Flu

Colds are always unpleasant and flu can be very serious. Whatever their severity, however, colds and flu can exacerbate chronic problems such as asthma, allergies and heart disorders and, of course, they can affect sleep. This may be partly due to the infection itself, or to any medication taken to fight it.

So, at the first hint of a cold or flu, snap into action:

- Practise GB (5 mins) + SB (20 mins) + GB (5 mins) several times a day.
- Reduce your food intake – there is often a natural loss of appetite anyway.
- Increase body temperature and do not attempt to bring it down using an aspirin or similar medication, unless you have a very high fever.
- Increase your cortico-steroids if you take these for asthma, allergies, emphysema, arthritis or systemic disorder.
- Use MP if your nose is blocked.
- Do not take antibiotics – your own immune system should fight the bacteria – unless your condition is

getting considerably worse. Antibiotics are useless against flu unless there is another infection present.

Depression

Depression is one of the most serious psychological causes of sleepless nights. It can take years to treat it, with heavy doses of drugs and no guarantee of success. Sufferers are record-holders among the short sleepers of the world, and it is not uncommon to attribute depression to lack of sleep, which is why many doctors try to address the sleep problem as a way of tackling the depression.

Let's look at it from a different perspective however: perhaps short sleep is the body's defence mechanism against depression. Longer sleep would slow down metabolic processes and increase hyperventilation. Perhaps also the body tries to stay awake because dealing with problems subconsciously, i.e. during sleep, is too destructive for the mind. Modern orthodox medicine does not take this 'defence mechanism' idea into account, and tries to improve sleep by lengthening it.

Sufferers from depression often find that, while falling asleep is not actually a problem, their sleep is short and shallow with lots of dreams and awakenings. As we have seen, one way to deal with improving the quality of sleep is to go to bed only when you are really sleepy.

Physical exercise is known to be helpful in the battle against depression. As well as this, a useful technique to try whenever you feel a bout of depression looming is as follows:

MP + SB (3-4 mins). Repeat.

ST JOHN'S WORT – A NATURAL ANTIDEPRESSANT

• In Germany St John's wort outsells Prozac by 20 to 1

St John's wort is an aromatic perennial herb that produces a yellow flower with five petals. It is native to Europe but may be found today almost worldwide thriving, as it does, in hostile terrain, in sandy or rocky soil. For more than 2500 years the flowers, unopened buds and the upper leaves have been ground up and used in herbal healing, and the plant was well known to Hippocrates, the father of medicine. It was used in ancient Greece to treat ailments ranging from snakebite to anxiety!

However, in the past 20 years or so, St John's wort has been rediscovered for its benefits in treating, most commonly, depression and, by extension, one of its most common symptoms, insomnia.

People who are depressed sleep fitfully and often wake up very early. For centuries St John's wort has been recommended as a sleep aid and recent scientific studies seem to back this up. According to these studies, the most notable effect of taking St John's wort is that it can increase slow waves during the deeper stages of sleep (see pages 12-14), and a deficit of deep sleep is a symptom of depression. This effect is also advantageous to older people whose sleep quality diminishes with ageing (see pages 122-123).

St John's wort used in conjunction with breath control techniques could be a recipe for success in treating depression-related sleep problems.

Note: Seek advice from your doctor or pharmacist before taking St John's wort, particularly if you are already taking any form of medication or oral contraceptive.

This should have an immediate effect and will nip a bout of depression in the bud if you catch it early enough. However, you should not use it more than 3-4 times a day. If you do feel you need to do it more often, your depression may need the personal attention of a Breath Connection practitioner. Do not be afraid to make contact.

Some doctors and alternative health practitioners prefer a nutritional approach to depression, which includes supplementing the diet with vitamin B-complex, magnesium and herbs such as valerian. St John's wort (*Hypericum*) is also a popular treatment for sufferers from depression – particularly in Germany, where it is commonly prescribed by orthodox doctors as an antidepressant. It is said to have been in use for over 2500 years.

The results of a Japanese study focusing specifically on the stress-reducing properties of a herbal extract of *Garum armoricum*, suggest that this might well have a positive effect on depression. Sufferers who took part in the study experienced fewer mood swings and less in the way of anxiety.

It is certainly worth trying natural or herbal antidepressants, but in so doing it is important not to overlook one of the major contributory factors of depression, namely hyperventilation.

Eczema

Eczema is a chronic skin condition which causes itching and redness, most commonly on the cheeks in babies, the knees, elbows, wrists and ankles in children, and the sides of the fingers in adults. It affects approximately 20 per cent of the population and its cause is not clearly understood, although there are known to be hereditary and immuno-logical factors at work.

Orthodox medicine usually treats eczema with steroid creams. However this treatment is purely symptomatic and cannot hope to get to the root of the problem; it also has many side effects which include thinning of the skin, a tendency to bruise easily and poor healing of wounds. Other common recommendations to eczema sufferers include dietary advice, and the elimination of certain identifiable irritants such as detergents and house dust. Breath Connection techniques can be very successful in treating eczema in both adults and children.

Breath Connection Programme for Eczema in Children

- Tape your child's mouth at night.
- Ensure that your child does not sleep on his back.
- Eliminate chocolate, dairy foods and nuts from your child's diet, and try to ensure that he does not start overeating.
- Place olive or almond oil on affected areas of skin so that it 'breathes' less.
- During the day, encourage your child to breathe through the nose only.
- For symptomatic relief during the day your child should practise the 'steps' exercise (see Blocked Nose, pages 130-131) whenever he feels itchy and wants to scratch. At night try olive or almond oil as above, and try to use medical creams only when this does not appear to work.

Breath Connection Programme for Eczema in Adults

- Practise the following exercise whenever you feel itchy (but no more than six times a day):

MP + SB (1 min) + MP + SB (2-3 mins)

Consult a Breath Connection practitioner for further advice if this does not help.

There are a number of general measures which should be taken in conjunction with the above, as follows:

- Use olive or almond oil on the affected areas.
- Fasting for one or two days can be helpful as long as there are no contra-indications.
- You may need supplements of vitamins A, E and B-complex, zinc and selenium – check with your GP.
- Be extra vigilant with your breath control, particularly in emotional situations, as these can have a direct effect on your skin condition.

Emphysema

Emphysema sufferers (who tend to be aged around 50 or over) often experience sleep problems due to a misunderstanding of their disease and its treatment. Emphysema is considered in the medical world to be not only incurable, but also irreversible. This, however, need not necessarily be the case as we shall see.

Sufferers experience shortness of breath, considerably reduced lung capacity and damaged lung tissue, but what they don't realise is that their body is using reduced lung capacity to indicate that hyperventilation is actually the real enemy. What this means, of course, is that the nebulisers, oxygen, steroids and bronchodilators that so many sufferers regularly use, in fact make their condition worse, not better.

Here are some tips to help relieve symptoms, and therefore improve sleep:

- Reduce use of oxygen to a minimum, taking it only for a minute or two when you feel you really need to.
- Stop using nebulisers and try 'puffers' instead, taking one puff only at a time when breathless. A nebuliser gives you a far stronger dose than a puffer, so it is far easier to 'overdose' on one.
- If you are using steroids, make sure you are taking the correct dose.
- Gradually try to wean yourself off long-lasting bronchodilators.
- Start doing regular physical exercise, keeping your mouth shut when doing so. If you do some form of exercise already, try to build on this.
- If you practise any form of deep-breathing technique, STOP.
- Try the following breathing exercise:

  - Sit down comfortably and relax.
  - Place one hand on your chest, the other on your abdomen, and listen to your breathing.
  - Reduce your breathing by gradually taking in less and less air. Your hands should start to move less.
  - Practise the above four to five times daily, the last

time being just before bed, for three days.
- Then from Day 4 do as follows:
  - Sit down, relax and check your CP.
  - Practise SB (5 mins) + CP + SB (5 mins) + CP and so on for 30 minutes, three times a day – before breakfast, lunch or dinner, and bed.

You should feel a slight lack of air when you practise the above, and if you do it correctly your CP will gradually increase. This in turn will help your condition and with it your sleep.

Flu – (see Colds and Flu)

Heartburn

Heartburn (also known as gastro-oesophagal reflux or nocturnal reflux) is a burning sensation behind the breastbone, often caused by eating or drinking too much. It can also be exacerbated by smoking.

There is no specific Breath Connection treatment for heartburn. However, general awareness of your breathing at all times is advised, along with the following:

- Try to change your eating habits – for example, avoid large meals before going to bed, and target and eliminate those foods which you suspect induce the problem. Common culprits are cheese and rich or spicy foods.
- Avoid medical treatment of heartburn.
- Sleep on your left side.

- Tape your mouth at night.
- Increase your CP.

Hypertension

Hypertension presents us with a paradoxical problem. On the one hand sleep problems, in particular snoring and sleep apnoea, affect blood pressure but on the other hand, nearly all 'blood pressure drugs' have an adverse effect on sleep. If you take diuretics you will need to go to the toilet during the night, and beta-blockers and other similar drugs can cause sleep to be shallow, which means that your sleep loses its restorative effect. Added to this is the fact that drugs prescribed to treat high blood pressure do not address the cause of disease, but only the symptoms.

Successful treatment of high blood pressure through Breath Connection is a complicated and delicate process that should be undertaken under the guidance of a highly qualified Breath Connection practitioner. However, sufferers who wish to try some self-help remedies should find the techniques recommended for snoring (see page 56) and sleep apnoea (see pages 62-64) useful.

Hypoglycaemia

Hypoglycaemia (or low blood sugar) is a serious condition which can be life-threatening. Diabetics may become hypoglycaemic if they take too much insulin, if they have not eaten enough, or if they exercise too much. The problem can have an adverse effect on sleep if sufferers have to get up several times in the night to eat in order to prevent a drop in their blood sugar.

The orthodox medical treatment for this condition (insulin) is paradoxical since in many cases patients chronically overdose on insulin, which suppresses the body's own natural insulin production. Shallow Breathing (see page 41) can change the way in which the body's organs work, and this can be used to advantage by hypoglycaemics.

CASE HISTORY

Sylvia is a 48-year-old hypoglycaemic American woman. She was taking up to 30 vitamin and mineral supplements a day and eating at prescribed times to control her condition when she first came to see me. She even got up at night to eat. I managed to persuade her to eat only when she was hungry, and to change her breathing pattern, explaining that Shallow Breathing can change the way in which our organs work. After a couple of days she admitted to feeling better in herself, and said also that she was eating less frequently. She no longer had to get up in the night to eat. At the beginning of her treatment she did tend to oversleep (around 8-9 hours), but as she was so good with her antibreathing technique she soon reduced this to 6-7 hours. She also stopped taking the vitamin supplements!

Narcolepsy

This is a rare disorder in which sufferers feel sleepy during the day, to the extent that they may fall asleep while eating or talking, and during the night often experience frightening symptoms such as hallucinations. They may have episodes of paralysis (for up to a few minutes) on waking up.

The cause of the disease is unknown. However, if sufferers have a low CP they stand a good chance of showing some improvement with Breath Connection since their problem is likely to be hyperventilation-related.

The following exercises should be useful in dealing with narcolepsy. Try Exercise 1 3-4 times daily as a general measure, and Exercise 2 on a need basis, specifically when you feel sleepy:

1) CP + SB (10 mins) + MP + SB (10 mins) + CP
2) MP + SB (3-4 mins)

Nocturnal Eating Disorder

Nocturnal eating disorder is a condition in which sufferers go to the kitchen to eat in the middle of the night. They are either partly or fully asleep when they do so, and often know nothing of their actions until they get up in the morning and see the tell-tale signs in the kitchen or at their bedside. This disorder can be quite dangerous since sufferers are unaware of what they are eating or doing.

Breath Connection can be used to contain nocturnal eating disorders, particularly if hyperventilation lies at the root of the problem. However, each case needs to be individually assessed and it would therefore be best to seek advice from a qualified practitioner.

Palpitations

Sufferers from palpitations (abnormally fast heartbeats) find it very difficult to fall asleep. A quickened heartbeat is a normal reaction to physical, psychological or emotional stress: if your pulse is 60 (i.e. 60 heartbeats per minute at rest) it is to be expected that it would jump up to 120-150 when you run, drive a fast car or watch a thrilling movie, for example. Palpitations are, in fact, a manifestation of hyperventilation (you will experience the same effect if you sit in a chair and start deep, fast breathing), and should not normally last longer than a few minutes after you have stopped the activity in question.

The following technique is helpful in dealing with palpitations:

MP + SB (3 mins) + GB (5 mins). Repeat.

Practise this exercise whenever you feel that your heart is racing. If this is in the middle of the night, sit up before starting it. If you find that you are doing the exercise more than 4 times a day, consult a Breath Connection practitioner for further advice.

The pulse is a useful and sensitive indicator of the body's condition. In general (with the exception of a pathologically low pulse, as might be expected in chronic fatigue syndrome, or thyroid problems), the deeper you breathe, the higher your pulse rate. It can also go up after taking medication, after a meal, or as we have seen in response to physical movement or emotional stress. It is therefore worth heightening your awareness of your pulse so that you make an automatic mental connection with hyperventilation and take steps (as above) to deal with it.

Periodic Leg Movement Disorder

Sufferers from this disorder experience episodes of involuntary jerks of their legs at regular intervals – say, every 30 seconds or so – sometimes during the day, but mostly at night. The cause of the problem is unknown, but it is often associated with insomnia or excessive daytime sleepiness.

There is no specific treatment for periodic leg disorder but the following simple tips can make a difference:

- Tape your mouth at night, even if you think that you keep your mouth closed.
- Try to sleep in a foetal position, pulling your knees up close to your chest.
- Take 'contrast' showers, alternating hot and cold water and ending with cold, for a few days.
- Practise some form of light physical exercise (walking or swimming, for example) 2-3 hours before going to bed.
- Ensure that your diet is nutritionally sound and that it incorporates enough vitamins and minerals (magnesium is particularly important).
- Season your food with sea salt rather than table salt.
- Totally eliminate caffeine from your diet for at least 5-6 days.

Restless Leg Syndrome

Sufferers of restless leg syndrome (RLS), the cause of which is unknown, experience 'creepy-crawly' sensations in their legs when sitting, driving, and particularly when lying in bed. The condition induces discomfort and pain, a desire to stretch or move the legs, and difficulty in falling asleep.

Bearing in mind that a lack of CO_2 (due to hyper-ventilation) causes abnormal nervous impulses, and is therefore a major contributory factor in RLS, Breath Connection techniques can be very useful in controlling this unpleasant disorder. Try the following exercise whenever symptoms occur:

CP + SB (3 mins) + SBLA (3 mins)

If, after three weeks, there is no noticeable improvement it would be advisable to enrol in a Breath Connection workshop.

Stress

Stress is considered to be one of the most common and serious causes of insomnia, but it is also very frequently misunderstood. Contrary to popular belief, we do actually need a certain amount of stress in our lives – it functions as one of the most powerful survival mechanisms we have. It helps to mobilise our 'fight or flight' instinct by changing our heart rate, breathing pattern and various hormone levels.

However, unresolved stress can lead to distress, which is where the problems start. Anxiety and stress are major factors contributing to a vast number of illnesses. Being stressed out can upset digestion, raise blood pressure, alter the brain chemistry and trigger depression. It can also damage the immune system by upsetting our hormone balance. Any one of these conditions can, of course, take its toll on sleep.

CASE HISTORY

Jack, a 32-year-old businessman, originally came to me because he wanted to give up smoking – he smoked up to 20 cigarettes a day. However, it soon became apparent that his real problem was sleep, and the 'hangover' feeling he woke up with in spite of not drinking. He felt that he had to go to bed at 11 p.m., and if he missed that deadline he would have insomnia. He had tried sleeping pills, but they made him weak and drowsy during the day and did little for him at night. He had consulted his GP, who concluded that smoking was the root of the problem, so Jack cut down. This made no difference to his sleep problems though, and he started smoking more again.

When Jack came to me his CP was 12 seconds – he was breathing for five people. I explained that smoking was increasing hyperventilation, but that he was also hyper-ventilating as a result of feeling stressed about giving up smoking! Naturally his sleep suffered. Jack undertook the Insomnia Course (see pages 43-46) tailored to his own individual needs, he stopped sleeping on his water bed and cut down smoking again. The headaches were the first to go, then the fatigue and drowsiness disappeared, and Jack developed a healthy sleeping pattern. After five months he had a CP of 35 seconds, had lost weight, and had far more stamina and energy.

The sleep-stress connection is something of a vicious circle: the more stressed you are, the more difficulty you have in sleeping, and the more tired you become, the less able you are to cope with stress. Research has also shown that stress affects the deepest and most restorative stage of sleep, compounding an already difficult situation.

However, given that stress provides the perfect conditions for hyperventilation, if we control our breathing, we should also manage to get the better of stress. The following exercise should be practised whenever you feel stressed; it is very powerful and results may be noticed immediately:

MP + SB (1-2 mins) + CP + SB (2-3 mins)

CHAPTER 9

The Way Forward: Success with Breath Connection

So far we've looked at how we sleep, why we sleep, why we may not sleep, and above all, how to improve our quality of sleep. We've seen that no matter what the illness or condition is that affects our sleep, hyperventilation is nearly always the root cause and Breath Connection the key to solving the problem. But now let's take a look at some hard facts in an assessment of Breath Connection's success with various problems.

Insomnia

Success rate: 95-98 per cent

Insomnia, as we have seen, is not a disease in itself, but is usually a symptom of another underlying problem. Whatever that problem, whether it's asthma, emphysema, allergies, depression, arthritis, hypertension or one or more of many other conditions (see Chapter 8), hyperventilation is likely to be at work. If you attempt to address your insomnia directly, using herbal remedies, sleeping pills or hypnosis, for example, your sleep may improve – and probably in the short-term only – but you may well feel drowsy during the day or have headaches in the mornings. The excellent success rate of Breath Connection in the treatment of insomnia is explained simply by the role of hyperventilation in almost any sleeping problem.

Snoring

Success rate: practically 100 per cent

Nearly everybody who has complained of a snoring problem has succeeded in doing away with it using Breath Connection techniques. Success for anybody of any weight or height, no matter what the shape of their nose or the configuration of their throat, is guaranteed by three things: a closed mouth, sleeping on the left side and breathing more shallowly. In fact, breathing less is the deciding factor, while a closed mouth and sleeping on the left side are complementary techniques. The simple fact is that if your breathing is shallow and gentle, you will be physically unable to snore since you will not produce enough airflow to create a snoring sound. See also Chapters 3 and 4.

Sleep Apnoea

Success rate: 80-90 per cent

Sleep apnoea is a natural extension of snoring, and as such can be readily and successfully treated through Breath Connection. However, the drop in the success rate figures is caused by long-time CPAP pump users (see page 58), since it can be very difficult to reverse the negative effects of these machines. Not only do the machines not treat the problem, they actually increase hyperventilation, so the longer patients have been using them, the harder it is to undo the damage.

Nightmares

Success rate: practically 100 per cent

Nightmares are a manifestation of acute hyperventilation which stimulates the nervous system and also reduces the level of oxygen in the brain, causing it to create frightening images. Breath control can deal with this effectively and also very quickly – results can normally be seen within a few days. There is also a similar rate of success with 'heavy' dreams, which are a simplified version of nightmares. See also Chapter 4.

Jet Lag

Success rate: practically 100 per cent

Jet lag is a part-physiological, part-psychological problem. The physiological aspect stems from hyperventilation, as well as a physical reaction to changes in climate, noise, a different bed, and various other irritants. The psychological factor is caused by the feeling that you have been 'robbed' of so many hours' sleep (the 'want' versus 'need' syndrome – see Chapter 2), making you feel angry and stressed. Breath control solves both problems by decreasing hyperventilation and recharging your body through a shorter, but deeper sleep. See also Chapter 6.

The Way Forward

So, where do we go from here?

The first thing to do is to stop listening to traditional advice like 'Make sure you get adequate sleep each night', 'Establish a regular sleep schedule', 'Unbroken sleep is essential' and 'Always make up for lost sleep'. We've seen that all of these popularly held beliefs are misconceptions, and that they do not play a part in solving sleep problems.

Similarly, there are various recommendations as to what you should avoid: alcohol, tobacco, tea, coffee and telephone calls within an hour of going to bed; eating a meal within three hours of going to bed; watching TV in bed less than an hour before going to sleep; fatty foods, red meat, salt, sugar, spicy food and greasy, protein-rich food; worry and stress; disturbances from light, noise and pets, and so on.

Of course, some of these bans make sense, and others less so, but why not trade these small bans for one big one: hyperventilation. If you establish a physiologically normal breathing pattern and gain control over your breathing, you will be better equipped to judge for yourself just what is good or bad for you. For example, if you are eating the wrong food, your breathing will get deeper, and you will be able to read the signals and address the problem. Likewise, you may sense changes in your breathing when you finish a second cigarette, or drink a second or third cup of coffee. The signals have always been there, of course, but Breath Connection teaches you how to recognise and deal with them. The excellent success rate of Breath Connection in the treatment of insomnia is explained simply by the role of hyperventilation in almost any sleeping problem. And when you get into bed and watch TV or read a book, your breathing will tell you whether or not you are setting yourself up for a bad night.

So let's work on the one big ban, which should be enough to look after your sleep and, in most instances, your general health and well-being too. Breath control may not always be easy to learn, particularly since for many of us it means giving up some firmly held beliefs and ideas, but once mastered it will set you up for a lifetime.

Commonly Asked Questions

Q Is it true that sleep-deprived people are more vulnerable to infections because their immune system is weakened?
A Numerous studies on rats, mice and rabbits appear to have proved that lack of sleep does weaken the immune system. However, let's take a closer look at what really happens.

The animals used in such studies experience high levels of stress. They are taken out of their environment and then in order to deprive them of sleep, they are forcibly kept awake. They may be pushed, shaken, given electric shocks or have water poured either on them or on the floor of their cages. It would therefore seem that stress, together with infection, and not just infection alone, could in fact kill them.

Q Do 'short' sleepers experience a sort of 'mental fatigue' during the day, making them slow in decision-making?
A A person who sleeps less due to stress, a family crisis, pain or illness may well find their judgement and decision-making powers impaired. This is because their lack of sleep is caused by hyperventilation which means that their brains are being deprived of oxygen. They cannot be expected to function to their best ability.

However, a person who breathes correctly may sleep fewer hours yet sleep better, and will feel fully restored and energised during the day.

Q Is there any truth in the theory that switching off the TV and reading a boring book before bed will help you to get to sleep?
A If what you want is to sleep more, then it may well be a good idea: engaging in boring activities dulls the mind and makes you feel sleepy. Hypnotists use a similar technique to induce a trance-like state. However, more sleep is not what you should be aiming for.

Q Is it normal and healthy to remember dreams? Should I worry that I don't?
A While it is normal to have dreams, it is not necessarily healthy to remember them; if you do it means that you are not sleeping deeply enough. Although dreams can often be funny, quite surprisingly and even bizzarely entertaining and reassuring in some ways they do not have any physiological value, and the fact that you remember them is an indication of hyperventilation and shallow, unhealthy sleep.

Q My son snores and we have been advised by our GP to have his tonsils and adenoids removed? Should we go ahead? Is this a good idea or is there in fact a better solution?
A Adenoids, as well as polyps, are in fact a natural defence mechanism against hyperventilation since they help reduce the amount of exhaled air (in other words CO_2) and narrow the nasal passages. It would therefore be a mistake

to remove them. Instead, by breathing less and 'listening' to your body's signals, you will help your body to shrink the adenoids, precluding any need for surgery. To solve your son's problem, therefore, you should help him to practise the Breath Connection techniques given for asthma (see page 116) – in fact, this problem is known to Breath Connection practitioners as 'asthma in the nose'.

Q As the mother of a two-year-old child who suffers from asthma, I am scared to tape his mouth at night.
A Don't be scared. Do it. But sit near him and watch him all night for the first night. Then you will see that he sleeps better and has fewer asthma problems in the morning. In fact, you should be scared to *let* him breathe through his mouth, no to prevent him doing it.

Q My chiropractor has recommended that I sleep on my back, with my arms and legs stretched, as this is best for my spine. Would you agree?
A No. Your chiropractor has not taken hyperventilation into account when advocating that you sleep on your back. Hyperventilation can create metabolic disturbances in the body which may result in hormonal imbalances, osteo-porosis and arthritis, which can cause back and muscular pains. So sleeping on your back may in fact contribute to your back pain rather than alleviate it.

Q Is it true that snoring at night is harmless if you do not feel drowsy during the day, and you do not have heart or blood pressure problems?
A No. There is no such thing as harmless snoring. Snoring and hyperventilation go hand in hand, so the seeds of

health problems are already sown, and the symptoms will inevitably follow, whether sooner or later.

Q If I sleep fewer than my usual seven hours one night, should I try to catch up the next night?
A Don't be concerned about sleeping too little. If you look after your body by practising your breathing techniques, your body will look after you, and you will find that from seven hours sleep you will come down to six or even five hours quite comfortably. Breath Connection will enable you to sleep deeper and shorter with no negative effects.

Q I have heard that sleep disorders can be fatal. Is this true?
A This is a classic example of modern medicine's misunderstanding of sleep disorders. You may well read studies showing that disrupted sleep intensifies heart and circulation problems, or that chronicly poor sleepers will die earlier, or that there is a higher incidence of stroke and heart attacks among poor sleepers. However, the misunderstanding lies in the fact that sleep – or lack of it – is not the culprit, and is only secondary to other problems, just as a temperature is secondary to an infection.

Q I love swimming, but find it impossible to swim with a closed mouth. Can it be done?
A It is perfectly safe and healthy to swim with the mouth closed, albeit much more difficult than swimming with an open mouth, and it does therefore require practice. Start with either the breast-stroke or by swimming on your back in order to get used to it, and swim slowly at first. Keep

your head above the water even if this slows you down. After a swimming session you should sit down and practise the Shallow Breathing technique for 10-15 minutes for maximum benefit.

Q I was always taught to breathe in sharply through my nose when I run, and out through my mouth, saying 'ha' as I do so. Is that correct?

A No. You should train yourself to run breathing only through the nose, and with the mouth shut. It is not easy, but it can definitely be done. However, you will probably need to increase your CP in order to achieve it.

Q My son suffers from cystic fibrosis. He has to practise deep-breathing exercises and a coughing technique with a physiotherapist to cough up his sticky mucus three times a day. How can Shallow Breathing help him?

A Shallow Breathing can help to make sticky mucus thinner, so that it comes out more easily on its own without the coughing technique.

Q I live on my own and am afraid to tape my mouth in case my nose gets blocked up and, with nobody around to help, I suffocate.

A Don't be afraid. The tape is not an enforced gag and if at any stage you find it difficult to breathe through the nose, or you feel panicky, simply rip it off. In time you will get used to it, and eventually you will keep your mouth closed without needing to tape it. Also, remember that by breathing through the nose you reduce hyperventilation, which in turn will help to prevent your nose from getting blocked up.

Q Is it possible to hyperventilate through the nose?
A Yes. If you breathe deeply and heavily through the nose you are hyperventilating, although not as much as you would be doing by breathing deeply through the mouth.

Q It sounds as if the Breath Connection method is a sort of panacea for all disorders.
A It may seem like that, but it is not true. We only use it to treat disorders that are related directly (like panic attacks or asthma) or indirectly (like arthritis or haemorrhoids) to hyperventilation. This means about 200 diseases and symptoms out of about 30,000 known to modern medicine. Or, to put it another way, about 0.6 per cent of all known diseases.

But that 0.6 per cent 'covers' about 80 per cent of the population because it includes the most common diseases. The power of breath, whether destructive or healing, should not be underestimated. It takes just 1-2 minutes of hyperventilation for even an Olympic champion to develop dizziness, palpitations, pins and needles and a drop in oxygen levels. In 15-20 seconds a severe asthmatic would develop a cough, wheezing, breathlessness or tightness in the chest. Those who are predisposed to problems connected to the heart or circulation will experience angina or a significant rise in blood pressure in about a minute. Such is the power of destructive deep breathing.

On the other hand it takes just 1 minute to unblock a chronically blocked nose, to stop arthritic pain, a headache, a coughing fit, anger, irritation, a panic attack, an eczema itch and dizziness using the Breath Connection method – if you know how.   ·

Theoretical Understanding behind the Breath Connection Method

The Breath Connection Method (The Buteyko technique) represents a development of the hyperventilation syndrome theory. This theory is based on the contemporary understanding of the immense biological role of the carbon dioxide gas in the human organism.

The human metabolism developed in the ancient geological eras when carbon dioxide in the air and water was represented in tens of percent. It is probably due to this factor that a concentration of CO_2 (7 per cent approx.) must be an essential condition of each human cell for it to sustain all the normal pathways of the biochemical processes.

The problem faced by the evolving human organism has been the depletion of CO_2 in our atmosphere from the tens of percent of ancient eras to the current level (1982) of 0.03 per cent. Human evolution has dealt with this dilemma by creating an autonomous internal air environment within the alveolar spaces of the lungs. These alveoli contain around 6.5 per cent of CO_2, quite a contrast to the surrounding air. The gaseous mix in the womb is also an interesting indicator of the ideal human environment. Here there exists between 7-8 per cent of CO_2. Professor Buteyko was asked to speak on this subject at the World Congress of Biochemistry which took place in Moscow in 1972.

Current Physiological Understanding

1. CO_2 is, through the conversion into carbonic acid, the most important buffer system in the body's regulation of its acid-base balance (acid-alkali balance). A low level of CO_2 may lead to alkalosis. If the level of CO_2 lowers to below 3 per cent shifting the pH to 8 then the whole organism dies.

2. A low level of CO_2 causes a displacement of the oxyhemoglobin dissociation curve, thereby not allowing correct oxygenation of the tissues and vital organs (the Bohr effect).

3. Poor oxygenation leads to hypoxia and a whole gamut of medical disorders.
4. CO_2 is a smooth muscle vessel dilator. Therefore a shortfall of CO_2 causes spasms of brain and bronchus tissue, etc.
5. Hyperventilation causes a progressive loss of CO_2. The higher the breathing, the lower the CO_2 level.
6. CO_2 is the catalyst to the body's metabolic processes, playing a vital role in biosynthesis of amino acids and their amides, lipids and carbohydrates, etc.

Through an understanding of current physiology we should begin to see the links between CO_2 and oxygenation of the body, and CO_2 and disease. It is clear that a deepening of the breathing does not mean an increase in oxygen uptake. On the contrary it means a decrease in oxygenation which leads to hypoxia, an imbalance in the acid-alkali balance and cell spasms.

The fifth point of physiological understanding explains the destructively poisonous influence that hyperventilation has on the organism. It shows us clearly (in conjunction with the other points) that over breathing leads to an imbalance in the body and a general deterioration of health.

The Dangers of Hyperventilation

The term 'hyperventilation' should be clearly defined. It is not reserved only for the most extreme and visible cases. Hyperventilation simply means an increase in the function of the lungs above the normal recommended amount. The significance of Buteyko's discoveries hinge on the diagnosis of what Buteyko termed "hidden hyperventilation", that is long term overbreathing that is not clearly visible in the patient.

If a patient hyperventilating at 30 lt/min can receive disastrous physical repercussions in the very short term, then it should be understood that overbreathing at 5-10 lt/min will have equally dire consequences over the long term. The average asthmatic overbreathes between 3-5 times the recommended amount, sometimes more.

The detrimental influence of deep breathing on the organism is a direct result of the creation of a CO_2 deficit. This has been proven by many experiments, starting with the work of the well-known physiologist, Dr D Henderson, in 1909. In his experiments, animals were mechanically induced to deep breath and died as a result.

Acid-Alkali Balance

Through its conversion into carbonic acid, CO_2 is the most vital player in maintaining the body's acid-base balance. Lowering CO_2 in the lungs by deep breathing shifts the body's pH towards alkalinity, which changes the rate of activity of all body ferments and vitamins. An alkaline system is more susceptible to virus and allergies. The shift in the rate of metabolic regulatory activity disturbs the normal flow of metabolic processes and leads to the death of the cell. As mentioned before, if the level of CO_2 is lowered below 3 per cent, shifting the pH to 8, the whole of the organism dies.

Hyperventilation, Disease and Modern Medicine

Symptoms of various combined disturbances in the organism of a deep-breathing person are exceptionally diverse. The traditional methods of disease analysis have resulted in various symptoms of overbreathing: (bronchospasms, heart muscle spasms, increased or decreased arterial pressures, and fainting spells with convulsions) being called separate illnesses such as bronchial asthma, stenocardia, hypertension and allergies, etc. All these 'separate illnesses' lead to complications, sclerosis of the lungs and vessels, myocardial infarcts and strokes.

The theory of the diseases of deep breathing has previously been presented in a lecture: 'On Discovery of Deep Breathing Being the Principal Reason for Allergies, Sclerosis, Psychosis, Tuberculosis, Pre-cancerous Conditions and Other Symptoms of Disease.'

In that lecture Professor Buteyko mentioned that his discovery is not only represented in the method of treatment of the diseases, but in the exposure of their causes. Professor Buteyko believes that modern medicine has slipped to the levels of blind empiricism. This appears to have happened because attempts to find the causes of diseases such as asthma, stenocardia and hypertension, etc., have been fruitless, there-fore an important principle of medicine is being trampled on. The very principle upon which the Buteyko philosophy is based: 'Having not found the reason of the disease, the physician has no right to treat the patient. Only having discovered the reason for the disease is it possible to guarantee the recovery.'

Modern medicine, as it stands at the moment, has either stopped looking for the causes of asthma, stenocardia, hypertension, etc., or it has a false impression of their causes. That is why these diseases continue to remain incurable. Through understanding 'trigger factors' we can only hope to treat the problem symptomatically. Only through the understanding of the cause of the disease can we hope to cure.

It is evident, through Professor Buteyko's research, that deep breathing is directly linked to at least 150 diseases. Buteyko has conducted an immense synthesis of diseases and has found that problems such as asthma, hypertension, stenocardia, myocardial infarcts, strokes, haemorrhoids and eczema, amongst others, are all symptoms of the imbalance created by deep breathing. In cases where Buteyko's patients had these diseases, they have all been cured. The

Buteyko theory cites that these diseases are the body's defence mechanisms against the excessive loss of CO_2 through overventilation.

The Nervous System

The lowering of CO_2 in the nerve cells heightens the threshold of their excitability, alerting all branches of the nervous system and rendering it extraordinarily sensitive to outside stimuli. This leads to irritability, sleeplessness, stress problems, unfounded anxiety fears and allergic reactions, etc. Concurrent with this, the breathing centre in the brain is further stimulated thereby causing a further loss of CO_2. In this way another vicious cycle had commenced.

The Causes of Deep Breathing

Having touched directly on the physiological problems of hyperventilation, and the resulting 'blowing off' of CO_2, an obvious question arises: What is the cause of deep breathing itself? What is hyperventilation a consequence of?

There are several factors known to induce deepening of the breath. The most important factor, in Buteyko's opinion, is the propaganda of the usefulness of deep-breathing. The contemporary man starts to be taught to breathe deeply even before he is born, when his mother is sent for sessions of deep-breathing exercises during her pregnancy. Often the newly born is encouraged to increase his breathing by having his little arms raised and lowered. And so it follows, in kindergartens, schools, armies and sport, etc. Deep breathing is encouraged without any scientific basis.

There are other factors as well – overeating, especially of animal protein (fish, chicken, eggs, milk and, naturally, meat) sharply increases breathing. It should be noted that the animal products increase the breathing more than plant products; cooked food more than raw.

Another factor deepening the breath is a state of limited mobility, lack of physical work or activity and idleness. Physical activity encourages the release of CO_2 from the cells, increasing its levels in the body. The breath is deepened by hydrodynamics, by bed-rest regimes, by prolonged horizontal positions (especially lying on the back) and by prolonged sleep. Recommendations for longer periods of sleep and even sleep therapy have never cured anybody. Most attacks of epilepsy, asthma, myocardial infarction, strokes and paralysis etc. occur towards the end of sleep, around 5 a.m.

Further factors deepening the breath are the various emotions (either positive or negative), stress, heat and stuffy environments. And conversely calmness, temperance and low temperatures aid shallow breathing.

The Aim of the Buteyko Method

The aim of the Buteyko method is to correct the patient's breathing pattern, that is to recondition the breathing pattern to internationally recommended physiological levels. Through this process the shortfall of CO_2 is also rectified. The Buteyko process is completely safe and drug free.

In contrast to the dangers of low CO_2, if the depth of breathing is decreased to below normal and the level of CO_2 in the organism is above normal by 0.5-1.0 per cent, there are no negative symptoms manifested. On the contrary, those afflicted with the heavy consequences of deep breathing, e.g. bronchial asthma, stenocardia and hypertension, develop symptoms of super-endurance with higher than normal levels of CO_2. The Buteyko clinics have been regularly observing this for the second decade now. It is evident that decreasing the depth of breathing does not result in any kind of undesirable occurrences.

What is the normal or correct amount of air we should be breathing? This varies from person to person but should be an average of 3-4 lt/min.

BIBLIOGRAPHY

Adverse Drugs Reaction Bulletin, August 1994.

Ball, N. & Hough, N. 1998. *The Sleep Solution* (Vermilion)

Buckman, D. D. 1999. *The Complete Guide to Natural Sleep*

Chopra, Deepak. 1996. *Restful Sleep: the complete mind/body program for overcoming insomnia* (Crown)

Clark, Susan. 1999. 'How Warm Milk and a Hot Bath Can Help You Sleep' (*The Times*, 16 November)

Clayton, Dr Paul. 1994. *Stop Counting Sheep, Self-help for Insomnia Sufferers* (Headline)

Coren, S. 1999. *Sleep Thieves.*

Courtenay, Anthea. 1990. *Natural Sleep, How to Beat Insomnia Without Drugs* (Thorsons)

Douglas, Jo & Richards, Naomi. 1984. *My Child Won't Sleep* (Penguin)

Flaws, Bob. 1997. *Chinese Medicine Cures: Insomnia* (Foulsham)

Folgering, H. & Snik, A. 1988. 'Hyperventilation Syndrome & Muscle Fatigue' (*Journal of Psychosomatic Research*, Vol. 32)

Gayrard, P., Orehek, J., Grimaud, C., and Charpin, J. 1975. 'Bronchoconstrictor effects of a deep inspiration in patients with asthma' (*American Review of Respiratory Diseases*).

Goldberg, B. 1998. *Alternative Medicine Guide to Sleep Disorders* (Future Medicine Publications)

Guilleminault, C. 1987. *Sleep and its Disorders in Children* (Raven Press)

Haldane, J. S. & Priestley, J. 1935. *Respiration.*

Hames, Penny. 1998. *NCT Book of Sleep* (Thorsons)

Innocenti, Dr. 1986. 'Chronic Hyperventilation' in *Text Book for Physiotherapists*

Johnson, T. S. & Halberstadt, J. 1992. *Phantom of the Night: overcome sleep apnoea syndrome and snoring – win your hidden struggle to breathe, sleep and live* (New Technology Publishing)

Katzenstein, Larry. 1998. *Secrets of St John's Wort* (Hodder & Stoughton)

Kirsta, Alix. 1986. *The Book of Stress Survival* (Gaia)

Lewis, K. H. & Howell, J. B. L.1986. 'Definition of the HVS.' (*Bulletin of European Physiopathology and Respiration* 22: 201)

Lipman, D. S. 1997. *Snoring from A to Zzz: proven cures for the night's worst nuisance* (Spencer Press)

National Commission on Sleep Disorders Research. 1994. *Wake Up America: a national sleep alert* (US Government Printing Office)

Naughton, M., Benard, D., Rutherford, R. & Bradley, T. 1994. 'Effect of continuous positive airway pressure on central sleep apnoea and nocturnal PCO_2 in heart failure' (*American Journal of Critical Care Medicine*, 1509, 1598-1604)

Sears, M. et al. 1987. '75 deaths in asthmatics prescribed home nebulisers' (*British Medical Journal*, 294)

Stalmatski, Alexander. 1997. *Freedom from Asthma* (Kyle Cathie)

Straten, Michael van. 1993. *The Good Sleep Guide* (Kyle Cathie)

Tobin, M. J. et al. 1963. 'Breathing patterns, diseases subjects.' (*Chest*, 84:287-94)

Utley, M. J. 1995. *Narcolepsy: a funny disorder that's no laughing matter*

West, B. 1995, 4th edition. *Respiratory Physiology* (Williams & Williams)

Wolf, Dr Danny. 1991. *Getting Your Child to Sleep* (Bellew Publishing)

www.sleepfoundation.org
www.allkids.org
www.keytodepression.com
www.excelnutrition.co.uk
www.sleepmed.com
www.prescriptionforsleep.com

INDEX